The Funny thing About Bladder Cancer

Guy B. Wheatley

DEDICATION

For Sharon, the center of my universe.

Thanks to friends and family who encouraged me to keep writing. Thanks to the doctors and nurses who kept me alive.

I wish to dedicate this effort to all cancer survivors, their families, and to the dedicated medical professionals who fight this destroyer of families. I am grateful for your courage and perseverance.

Contents

DEDICATION......................................iii

Confirmation..1

The Beginning....................................10

The First Doctor Visits......................22

The Bad News....................................31

The hospital.......................................44

After The Surgery.............................51

Leaving the Hospital.........................62

The First Excursions.........................71

Life Without Tubes...........................81

Life After Cancer..............................90

ABOUT THE AUTHOR...................94

CONFIRMATION

I wasn't surprised to see an attractive young woman step into the exam room. I knew that before the doctor came in, somebody else would first take my blood pressure and ask all of those personal questions again. She quickly finished that then said. "OK, let me explain what is going to happen."

Now I was sitting in a urology clinic to have the doctor shove a camera into an orifice one would not normally expect to accommodate a camera. I pretty well knew what was going to happen. But she had a job to do, and far be it from me to thwart the industry of a dedicated professional, so I let her continue.

"OK Mr. Wheatley," she began. "You'll need to drop your trousers and underwear to your ankles, then lay face up on the exam table. You can cover yourself with this sheet. I'll step out until you're ready. Then I'll prepare the area with betadine and inject lidocaine into your urethra."

I remember seeing her lips continue to move after that last sentence, and I vaguely remember sounds like human speech, but there was nothing in the form of information

1

reaching my brain. It was too busy screaming inside my skull, "WHO'S going to do WHAT to WHOM?

I felt strange enough even acknowledging to such a young woman that I possessed those parts. I thought I'd taken quite a step being able to discuss their function in a small, dispassionate and academic way. But now I was learning that she would be the one to actually treat them. Fortunately, this was such an emotional overload that I just went numb and was paralyzed into inaction. Otherwise, I'm sure I would have run from the room. My brain finally cooled down some and I again began to discern actual communication in the sounds she was making.

"I'll step out now. You get ready on the table," she told me. Then true to her word, she left the room. I don't know why. It's not like I was going to grow different parts after laying down. She wasn't going to see anything while I was standing that she wasn't going to be actually handling a few minutes from now. I dropped my pants, then lay back on the table clutching the sheet like a life preserver. A second later there was a quick rap on the door and she called, "Ready?"

"Yes ma'am," I timidly responded.

She stepped around the table pulling on a pair of latex gloves, then lifted the sheet. And there I lay, sheet up, pants down, while a woman younger than my daughter surveyed the area. I can assure you that nobody would have been the least bit impressed with anything found there at that moment. I couldn't have been less impressive sitting in a tub of crushed ice. I consoled myself with the thought that this would not be the first time she had examined a scared to death, little piece of malfunctioning equipment, desperately trying to hide. Nor was it likely to be the last, and with the next victim, I'd hopefully become just one in a forgettable procession.

At this point, I expected her to go into cold, clinical, robot mode, but that's not what happened. I remember when my father-in-law passed away. He had been confined to the hospital for quite a while. I have twin nieces, about my daughters age. One of them became a nurse. I remember being fascinated, watching the girl I still thought of as a child switch to nurse mode. Suddenly, where one of my daughter's play mates had stood, was a competent, professional nurse. But in this case, mingled with the professional care, was the love for a beloved grandfather. It was an incredible mix of confident, competent medical care delivered with a tenderness that exceeds my ability to put into words. I remember thinking how fortunate Mr. Greenhill was to have her there.

That memory came to me in this moment because this young woman was doing almost the same thing. I don't remember any of the actual words she used. I don't remember her tone of voice. I do remember her looking into my eyes as she asked how I was doing, or if I was hurting. That's odd, because I remember definitely planning to not make eye contact. In some way, she conveyed genuine concern with out demeaning pity. I would have been surprised for a seasoned nurse, calling on a long lifetime of experience to pull that off. How someone so young did it, I'll never know. But I don't have to understand it to be grateful for it.

She finished what ever it was she was doing, then gently replaced the sheet. "The doctor will be right in," she assured me. Unbeknownst to her, the doctor was tied up and would not be right in. As much as I wanted this over with, I dreaded what was to come too much to be able to wish he'd hurry up. As I lay there with conflicting emotions, another factor soon began to make itself apparent giving me cause to reconsider my strategy for that day.

I'd made the Seventy-four mile trip on this hundred-and-five-degree day by motorcycle. I had several reasons for that. One was gas. At three-and-a-half dollars a gallon, I saved quite a bit by taking the bike. Another reason was that I rarely pass up a chance for a ride. Unless there's a compelling reason to take a larger vehicle, I'll usually go on the bike. And finally, I don't know how many more rides I'll get to take. While I had not pulled that thought out and looked it over real close, somewhere in the back of my mind was the idea that I might not be able to ride much longer. So, a hundred-and-five-degrees or not, I'd taken the bike.

I'd been told to drink two quarts of water forty-minutes before my appointment. I filled up an insulated quart water bottle with crushed ice and water and slung it around my neck before heading out. By the time I got to Shreveport, it was empty. I checked in at the desk, then filled the bottle from a water fountain and drained it again. I did this three more times before finally being called to the exam room.

By the time I was making my way down the hall toward the exam room, my eyes were floating. I'm sure I'd sweated out a lot of water on my ride over, but that five quarts I'd downed in the last hour-and-a-half had apparently been more than enough to top me off. Now the excess was demanding release. I knew that I was going to be called upon to deliver a urine a specimen, so in just a few more minutes blessed relief would be at hand. Sure enough, the exam room shared a bathroom with another exam room. The lady who escorted me here instructed me to go inside and provide the sample. I quickly filled the thimble sized specimen cup, then began to seriously tax the clinic's sewerage system. I eventually finished and somewhat to my astonishment neither ruptured the pipes nor washed away the buildings foundation.

But shortly after leaving the rest room, I again felt the waters building. Absent from my previous narrative was that I made one more pit stop before dropping my trousers and laying on the table. I figured that would surely get me through the ordeal to come. And without the doctor's delay, it might have.

My kidneys, apparently excited by the sudden attention of a renal specialist, were determined to put on a good show. They were moving water at a rate that would have done Niagara Falls proud. My poor diseased bladder was much less ambitious. It was, in fact quite adamant in its displeasure. By the time the doctor arrived, there was no hope that I could make it through the exam. "Sorry doc," I said, " but I've got to go."

"That's alright." he assured me patiently. "You go ahead."

I slid from the table and modestly clutched the sheet around me as I shuffled to the bathroom, pants still around my ankles. I finished my business and returned to the exam room where the doc gave me an apologetic look and said, "I'm sorry, but we'll have to prep you again." The attractive young woman began pulling on another pair of gloves.

My doctor's name is Spinazze, pronounced Spin-oz-zee. For some reason, my brain insists on reading it spin-uh-zee. Every time I call the clinic or check in, I wind up stammering, "Spin uh, uh spin uh," until somebody would helpful offer "Spin-oz-zee?"

"Yes," I'd reply embarrassed. This guy has touched me in ways no other human has, including my wife. Under normal circumstances, dinner and a movie would be the minimum prerequisites for such contact. On second thought, make that jewelry. Expensive jewelry. You'd think I could at least remember his name.

I called upon a technique I'd learned in Dale Carnegie where you picture the person in an amusing situation with some mnemonic visual cue. In this case, I used my neighbors big black Labrador. Her name is Oz, but of course we all call her Ozzy. So I just pictured the doc, spinning like a ballerina holding a big black Labrador Retriever over his head. I figured the slippers and a tutu would have been overkill, so he was in scrubs in my mental image.

But standing at the end of the table now, he wasn't holding a dog. The object was black and knowing what he was about to do with it, it looked huge. It didn't look at all friendly. I laid back and looked at the ceiling, as he said something. I don't remember the exact words, but it was basically a warning that he was about to start and that I might feel a little discomfort. If one would describe being impaled on a Roman pike as a little uncomfortable, then yeah, I felt a little discomfort.

When the good Lord designed the particular passage that was presently being invading, it was his intention that it conduct only liquids -and those only in one direction. Now it was suffering a solid object traveling the wrong way, and it was not happy. It was lighting up my neural pathways letting me know that it was't happy. The doc apologized and assured me he was, "almost there." He then shoved another twenty or thirty feet of that thing into me. I felt a pounding in my skull that I'm sure was the end of the probe trying to exit the top of my head. He cranked it around a couple of times, then pulled it out and said, "OK, That's it." The whole ordeal lasted less than thirty-seconds. It was intense but it was thankfully brief.

The doc had filled my bladder with sterile water before inserting the camera so I now had to hit the restroom again. "You can use the sheet to clean yourself up," the doctor told me. "Then we'll talk." I found myself alone as he and the young lady left the room.

"Then we'll talk." I wasn't prepared for the impact those three words had. I wasn't sure I wanted to talk. My knees felt wobbly as I shuffled toward the bathroom one more time. Up until this point, I hadn't considered that he would have things to tell me after the examination. I had concentrated on the mechanics of the procedure to the point of ignoring the reason for it. With the exam complete, there was now nothing between me and the news to come. Suddenly having a camera shoved into such a small sensitive hole was no longer the scary part.

I tried to concentrate on removing the gelatinous goo covering my groin area. Most of it seemed to be a clear substance, but parts of it were streaked with a reddish yellow material which I assume was the betadine. The linen sheet was only smearing it into successively thinner layers. I just couldn't seem to get that last little bit off. My bladder insisted I was clean enough though, and it was time to take care of the sterile water the good doctor had filled it with.

Something interesting happened here. My bladder dumped about 50cc of sterile water, but my urethra somehow passed about a gallon-and-a-half of flaming acid. The shock that paralyzed my upper torso and constricted my throat turned what should have been a window shattering scream into a sickly gurgle. Struggling to retain consciousness, I recalled the doctor's warning that for the next day or two when I urinate, I might experience a little discomfort.

We had the talk after I got dressed. I've had several talks since then. They all sort of run together to the point I'm no longer sure when I was told what. As I left that day, I had an appointment to be back in four days for a day surgery where the doctor would go in through my urethra and remove a tumor he'd seen. If it was confined to the lining of my bladder, then they could remove it and that would be it. I'd be done. If during the surgery he discovered it had spread any further, then we'd talk about what came next.

Back on the Valkyrie headed for Texarkana, I had almost an hour-and-a-half ride to digest what had just happened to me. I may have fudged the speed limit a time or two hitting 80 mph or better as I circled around Shreveport on I-220. The furnace hot blast washing over me somehow felt good. For the next hour-and-a-half I was a biker again. The frailty I'd felt dropped away with a twist of the wrist. The 1500cc flat six engine howled my defiance through the six into six cobra pipes, and it seemed that surely not even the big C could catch me while mounted on my powerful phat lady. I knew it was only an illusion, but it was one I came to cherish more with each subsequent trip.

The roughly three hours I spent in transit on each trip gave me time to come to grips with what was happening, an opportunity to build some perspective and start coming to grips with it emotionally. Riding the bike has always been cathartic for me, and now the drone of the engine and the wind in my face helped calm the fear waiting in the wings for an unguarded moment to pounce.

THE BEGINNING

As I rode, I reflected on how I had come to this place in my life. May of 2011 was the beginning of a record hot summer in Texas. I spent the last week of that month camping at Dinosaur Valley State Park near Glen Rose. I just couldn't stay hydrated enough to knock what felt like a reoccurring bladder infection. The last contraction as my bladder emptied was becoming increasingly painful. What's more, I would feel as though I needed to relieve myself, even after urinating. I discovered that soft drinks made it much worse so I restricted myself to water.

Some time in early June, back at work only a few days, I dumped the first bucket of blood. I was on my way home, and decided to make the trip with an empty bladder. I stopped by the men's room before leaving the building. Standing at the urinal, something felt different. As the stream began, that too had a different sensation from anything I'd ever felt before. I glanced down to see an opaque, bright red stream splashing onto the porcelain.

"Well this certainly does not look like a positive development," I remember thinking. The stream finally slowed to a trickle, leaving the inside of the urinal stained pink from the splatter. It took several flushes before it was again white. But try as I may, I couldn't seem to shake that last crimson drop from myself. No matter how vigorous my efforts, one more drop would appear waiting to stain my underwear. I finally realized I was going to need a piece of toilette tissue, which meant a trip to a stall. Just as I turned away from the urinal, legs bowed to keep blood droplets off my pant legs, and with equipment still dangling from my open fly, the door burst open and a couple of guys from the pressroom came in. I was spared from a rather awkward scene by the fact that they were talking to each other and hadn't noticed me. I quickly twirled back to the urinal and with a sigh, I put every thing away and left. It didn't really matter. Within a couple of weeks, every piece of underwear I had would be stained.

I had my iPhone in my hand as I exited onto the back parking lot, and called my General Practitioner to make an appointment. It usually takes a week or so to get in so I was surprised to get an appointment for the next day. Flipping over to my calendar, I noticed that I had a chiropractor appointment for the same time. I made an executive decision and canceled the chiropractor appointment. I figured that until I knew why I had blood coming out of my pee-pee, I didn't need some guy twisting me up like a pretzel, twisting my innards, and cracking my bones.

By the time I submitted a specimen my urine looked clear again, but the lab detected blood in the sample none-the-less. The doctor suggested it could be a bladder infection and put me on antibiotics to see if that would clear it up. We scheduled an appointment for two weeks later. If there was still blood in the urine, he'd set me up with a urologists.

Throughout the next week and a half, I'd clear up for a couple of days, then go red for a day or two. A couple of days before my appointment, I called and told the doctor that I was still passing blood. He said he would have his staff go ahead and make an appoint for me with the plumber. A few days later, I got a call from Column and Carney. That call was as educational as it was shocking.

— — —

You could say my troubles with them started a couple of years before, with my attempt to stay healthy. In 2009 I'd been feeling a fluttering in my chest, almost like butterflies were flying around in there. I'd also turn beet red and my ears would feel hot. I'd get a deafening ringing in my ears. I was fifty-three at the time, almost the same age my father died of a massive heart attack. I don't want to come off here as a Nervous Nelly, but with that family history, I figured those symptoms deserved at least a look. My General Practitioner set me up for a Cardiolite Stress Test. This involves hooking me up to up several million wires, then having me lay on my back with arms over my head while balancing on a bench the same size as a two-by-four wall stud. The position they wanted was easily achievable by dislocating both shoulders, and forgoing breathing for the twenty-minute duration of the test. I was required to lay half in the maw of some machine that was spinning things around me while it decided whether or not to finish eating me. This was before the "Transformers" movie, but looking back, that machine must have been the inspiration for the giant robot that was sucking up all of the good guys.

Surviving the transformer, I was then dragged across the room to a treadmill. As the the test continued, the folks administering it would raise the upper end of the treadmill making me run up hill. They did this several times, increasing the angle to the point I would soon need spider powers to stay aboard.

Through out this test the specialist kept warning me not to pass out, to let them know if I was becoming too fatigued as they didn't want me fall off. I don't think they wanted me to be flung across the room while still wired to their rather expensive looking equipment, possibly pulling some of it along with me and damaging it. They scrutinized the machines I was wired to as I ran. They would mutter to each other, then check off items on a clipboard.

Some time during the test, they injected the radioactive marker. This is a completely safe substance, brought into the room in a lead cask and handled by the specialist, now wearing radiation shielding, as he holds it at a distance from himself with a pair of tongs. Somehow, the opening scene of "The Simpson's," with Homer at work came to mind. I don't recall a green glow. "You might feel a slight burning," I was warned as the completely safe radioactive substance was injected into my veins.

Hey, I'm getting radioactive stuff injected into me. As I recall Peter Parker became the Amazing Spider man in a similar fashion. Maybe I'd get spider powers and be able to stay on the treadmill after all. Sadly, eight years on, I still can't climb the side of a building.

I kept running. It became important to me to finish. To "pass the test." It seemed that I was trying to outrun heart disease, that by my endurance I could stave off bad news. I still had a few more minutes in me when they finally shut the thing down.

As I finished, the cardiologist looked at me and said, "The only other person to completely finish this was a marathon runner in here for a required physical. Why the heck did your doctor send you over here?"

It turns out the chest fluttering was due to esophageal spasms caused by acid reflux. The red face, blotching on my neck and chest, the burning and ringing in my ears, was a histamine flush. My problems were easily solved with Prylosec and Benadryl, my heart is in great shape. What a relief.

A few months later I was back in the doctors office for a leg injury. He had been telling me I needed to get a colonoscopy and brought it up again on this visit. I told him to go ahead and set it up.

I won't go into the details of this procedure because I don't remember them. My experience was drinking some nasty stuff the day before, wearing an embarrassing outfit the day of the procedure, laying on a table getting ready for it, then being told it was over with. As horrible as the expectation was, the experience was far easier than the Cardiolite.

The results came back fine and it appeared I was an exceptionally healthy individual. If I didn't live forever, it wouldn't be colon cancer or a heart condition that got me. Talking to Column and Carney in 2011 I considered the irony. If things don't go well, it's strange to think that what might get me was not reading my insurance policy.

The two tests were done several months apart, but in the

same year. My insurance company will only pay for one of these "elective" tests in a calendar year. They refused to pay for the colonoscopy. It looks like I owed $1,200 to the doctor and $1,200 to the lab. I set up payment schedules and started sending in checks. A short time later Column and Carney sent me a past due notice. I checked and found where I'd sent the checks to the lab. I called them and told them I'd been sending payments, and the lady said she'd make note of it.

This happened about twice more, with me calling them each time. I'd get the same result, with the lady apologizing and saying she'd make note of it. The bills from Column and Carney eventually stopped only to be replaced by a phone call from a collection agency. Needless to say, I was livid. When I told the guy I'd flippin well been sending payments in, he quizzed me about how they were made out, where and when I'd sent them. Yes. I'd been paying the lab, but I also owed the clinic for the use of its facilities. The total bill wasn't $2,400, but $3,600. My red face this time had nothing to do with a histamine flush. Subdued and chastised, I set up a payment schedule and started sending checks to Column and Carney's collection agency as well.

Fast forward now to a few days after my General Practitioner said he'd set up an appointment for me with a urologists. I get a call from Column and Carney telling me that my doctor wants to set up an appointment, however, I still have a balance with them of $350.00. The lady was very apologetic, but said their accounting department couldn't allow me to incur any more debt with them until I reduced the current balance, and that the $50 per month we'd previously agreed too wasn't sufficient. They wanted $100, down, and a $100 payment. The next payment would was due within a couple of weeks. So I was basically going to have to cough up $300 in a couple of weeks. Embarrassed that I was in such a financial bind, and stunned that I was being denied medical care, I told the lady I'd see what I could do and get back to her.

Reviewing my finances, I realized that my only hope of getting the money involved a ski mask, a hand gun and a liquor store. Ruling out that option, I took the only other course of action available to me. That was to pretty much just cross my fingers and hope it wasn't serious.

I would go a few days without seeing blood. I'd convince myself that it had probably been an infection after all and I'd finally gotten over it. Then the crimson tide would return. I'm not even an Alabama fan.

I'd try to convince myself that the relapse was due to some factor that I could control. I'd been raking leaves and gotten hot the day before, so maybe that was why the blood returned. On one occasion, I'd indulged in a favored soft drink, maybe that was the reason for the relapse. Maybe if I was careful to not get too hot, or to not drink soft drinks. Maybe if I'd wear purple polk-a-dots and hop in a clockwise circle on my left leg. Deep in my gut, I knew this was all superstitious nonsense, but I had to try something.

And then it got a little worse. One morning as I attempted to relieve myself I had difficulty getting the stream started. Just as I began to realize that something was blocking my urethra, it came loose and passed through, landing with a splat in the urinal. It was an oblong object, dark brown in color and covered in pits or small holes. It looked for all the world like a slice of liver. I'm not sure what shocked me more. The strange sensation of the thing passing through my penis, or the sight of some part of my innards laying there in the urinal.

As a hunter who's cleaned his own game, I've got a decent idea of what most critters, including humans, look like on the inside. I couldn't see a way a piece of liver could get into my bladder, so I quickly dismissed that as the potential source, but could it be a piece of a disintegrating kidney? I had to know. Bending close with my face almost in the urinal, I began to poke at the thing with something I picked up from the floor. I don't remember what my tool was, but it was stiff enough to use as a probe.

This was taking place in a restroom at work. It wasn't the same one I'd almost been caught exposing myself in earlier. This one was in the news room, the one the reporters used. I knew if somebody came in while I had my face inches from the porcelain, it was going to look strange. I didn't care. I needed to know just what the hell had fallen out of my body.

Probing away, I again called on my experience cleaning game and was able to identify the object. It was a blood clot. Not the hard kind that forms when exposed to air like you see on the outside of a wound or bandage, this was a gelatinous clot that forms immersed in liquid. The coloring and surface pitting was caused by the acidic environment where it formed in my bladder. Though that first one was by far the largest, it was not the last blood clot I would pass. They got to be quite common.

I was drinking a lot of water to keep myself flushed out, but this now caused me to have to go to the bathroom more often. I didn't want to have to explain the chunky blood in the bowl or urinal to a coworker. It's bad enough to have a problem like this. But if somebody started asking questions about what the doctor said, or what I was doing about it, it would get even more embarrassing. I didn't want to admit that I couldn't afford to go. I earned a decent wage, and should have been able to deal with this. I was in this boat as a result of my own irresponsibility. I didn't want to have to admit that, nor did I want to have to outright lie. The best way to handle this was to be sure the conversation never came up. I got quite adept at catching the restrooms unoccupied. I always had a piece of toilette paper in my pocket to wipe away any blood spatter. I was able to keep anybody at work from finding out.

There was one person I couldn't keep it from. About the time I found out I wasn't be going to see a specialist at Column and Carney, I had one of my longest clear stretches. So when my wife asked me about it, I honestly told her that it looked like the problem had cleared up. Later, when the blood came back, I just didn't mention it to her. I built a wall of denial, excusing every relapse as the result of some external factor that I would avoid in the future. As long as she didn't ask again, I wouldn't mention it. If she did, then that would be it. One thing I knew of an absolute certainty after thirty-two years of marriage was that I could not lie to her. Once she locked those lovely green eyes on me and asked a direct question, there was no chance of my deceiving her.

I've only lied to her a few times in our lives together, and I can say those were the result of my misguided macho attempts to spare her from some unpleasantness. But once her suspicions are aroused, I've never been able to pull off a lie. She can see right through me. So the goal was to not raise those suspicions. Unfortunately, every nocturnal trip to the bathroom was an opportunity for exposure. I was very careful to be sure there were no tell-tell red spots left in the toilet once I'd finished, but after several weeks one managed to elude me. She found it the next morning, and that was it.

I explained to her that I couldn't get in to see a specialist at Column and Carney, to which she said, "Well call the GP and have them set you up with somebody in Shreveport or Little Rock."

I'm sure it was an interesting image, me standing there in the bathroom early one morning in my blood stained underwear, blinking my eyes in the early morning light, and wondering just why that idea never occurred to me. I called my GP as soon as the office was open and soon had an appointment scheduled in Shreveport with Dr. Spin uh … Spin uh … uh, - a urologist.

Sharon asked if I wanted her to go with me. I was able to honestly say no. I was sure that this first visit would be a shake your hand, what seems to be the problem, type of meeting. Any tests would be scheduled for another visit. If she went with me, we'd go in the Caviler. If I went by myself, I'd take the Valkyrie. I love my wife with all of my heart and soul and treasure each moment spent with her. But not even her presence could make three hours in a caviler equal to three hours on a Valkyrie. Thank you sweetheart, but I'll just go by myself.

The first meeting went mostly as I expected, though there was one small surprise. I don't know why I didn't realize that a urologist was going to check me for testicular cancer, but of course he did. As I stood there pants down and arms up, the first small piece of my dignity got chipped away. I gave him a brief run down of what had been happening, He ask some questions and I answered. He then set me up to come back and have a cat scan of my bladder and kidneys. He also explained that he would run a camera into my bladder through the urethra to see what it looked like. Depending on what he found from these tests, we'd discuss the next course of action.

I headed home without any real information, but strangely relieved. Seeing the doctor and having tests scheduled gave me a sense of accomplishment. At least I was doing something now, I was fighting back. A source of stress I hadn't really known was there was suddenly gone. I called Sharon, as promised, before leaving. I gassed up, then enjoyed one of the most relaxed and leisurely rides I can remember in a long time.

Over the next four days a few things started to take shape in my mind. I knew we were in a tight spot financially. Even though I have insurance and long term disability, there would be deductibles and co-payments. We were living paycheck to paycheck. If this turned into some sort of extended treatment, I wasn't sure where the money would come from. We had enough assets to get us back on good footing, but they weren't liquid. It would take time to convert them to cash. But until then, things were tight and we were pinching pennies. As time went on, the financial pressure became more of a strain than the medical issue.

On the day I returned to Shreveport for tests, we decided for me to go by myself on the bike. Sharon asked me if I wanted her to go with me, but I again said no for several reasons. One was that if things got more serious, she'd need to get in all of the work time she could before having to take time off. Second, going by myself, I'd be on the bike and using less gas. Third, and strangely, the most important reason was that, even riding through a hundred-and-five degree weather, the time on the motorcycle was therapeutic. I was beginning to suspect that soon I might not be riding for a while. I didn't want to pass up any chance for time in the saddle.

Four days after the first visit, I found myself sitting in an exam room, waiting on the urologists to run a camera up my willy. I wasn't surprised to see an attractive young woman step into the exam room.

THE FIRST DOCTOR VISITS

The third trip would not be on the bike. My poor little urethra would again be invaded by unnatural forces, but this time it would be on it's own as I would be asleep. Because of the anesthesia I would be unable to drive myself home. Additionally, they insisted that I have somebody with me throughout the entire procedure.

"Who ever comes with you can't leave," they incessantly reminded me. "They will have to stay in the waiting room. And if they're not a family member, they'll need to be able to contact a family member." That sounded pretty intense for a routine test, but I decided not to probe their reasoning too deeply. I wasn't sure I'd like the answer, assuming I'd even get a real answer.

Sharon and I again talked about whether she should go. Unfortunately it was an especially rough day at the bank. The first and third of the month fell over the a weekend and the bank was unusually busy. She insisted that she would take off and go with me, but I knew that it would be an extraordinary burden on her coworkers. With all of the government checks coming out on the Friday, it would not be a good day to be down a worker. I pointed out that every thing would probably be fine, but if not, she might need the personal day she would have used later on. Reluctantly she agreed, and I asked my best friend to take me.

— — —

I hate to describe Charles as a "Biker buddy," because our friendship goes beyond that. But we did meet because of the bikes. I'd just bought my second motorcycle, a 1994 VF750 Honda Magna. I didn't know much about motorcycles at the time. I just knew that it looked cool, seemed to be in good condition, and was in my price range. And 750cc seemed like a logical step up from the 250 I'd been riding. I'd never heard of a Magna, and had no idea just what I was getting. The guy I was buying it from, went on and on about a V-4 and having shimmed the jets and other techie stuff that didn't mean much to me at the time. I just saw a pretty motorcycle that I could afford. I did remember his mentioning a website called MOOT, which stands for Magna Owners Of Texas, and telling me that there were a lot of people on the site who could give me help and advise about this particular motorcycle. Over the next couple of weeks I came to understand that this was not some little 750 I'd bought. The third generation Magna is a V-4, high revving power cruiser that can throw 85 hp into a

550 lb. platform. There were very few motorcycles of the day that could keep up with it. I was soon able to distinguish it from the multitude of V-twins roaring up and down the roads.

Sharon and I decided on fast food on the evening we meet Charles and Brenda. We'd taken the caviler and were still in the parking lot when I spotted and man and woman sitting on a motorcycle at a stoplight on Stateline avenue. I recognized the bike as a Magna.

"Hey, That's a Magna!" I hollered at the guy.

Without comment, he flipped on his blinker and looped around into the parking lot. He pulled up next to the Caviler and I noticed that one of his arms was bigger than both of mine together. As he stepped from the bike, I couldn't read his expression. It wasn't quite a scowl, but neither was it puppy dog friendly. As that massive right arm began to move, I almost dove under the car. But he extended a friendly hand, and as he shook mine he said, "Hi. Charles Otwell. You like Magnas?"

Over the next couple of years, Charles and Brenda would be come not only our motorcycle mentors, but our best friends as well. So when I needed somebody to take me to Shreveport for a day surgery, of course it was Charles. I picked him up at at four-thirty that morning and we headed out, me driving. We left early. I've always been like that, especially about something I dread. It's like I'm anxious to get it over with and try to rush it. Conversation on the way over was light. We chatted about the things we usually talked about. It was just a regular bull session of the kind we don't get enough of.

We got to Shreveport with almost an hour to spare. I suggested that we stop someplace and let Charles get some breakfast. He didn't want to eat in front of me since I couldn't, but I assured him that I would much rather sit in a restaurant than in the clinic parking lot.

I grabbed a table as Charles placed his order. The sun was now up but the sky still had that early morning cast. I watched the other patrons and tried to imagine what their day would hold. Almost everyone of them had coffee of some flavor. Some were getting breakfast. One man appeared to be in his mid-thirties. He was dressed in a neat white shirt with a tie. He was reading a newspaper as he sipped at his coffee. He had an air of bored routine about him that told me he was beginning another boring, ordinary day. Lucky bastard.

A commotion at the counter caught my attention, and I noticed a woman with two small children, all wearing coats. The weather this day didn't really justify coats of that weight. Nobody else was dressed so warmly. The kids were a boy and a girl close to the same age, I guessed to be about 6-years-old. They didn't seem to be fully awake yet, irritably pulling on each other, and answering the woman's questions with whining complaints rather than informative responses.

The woman, who I presumed to be their mother, was scrutinizing the menu board with an intensity that made me believe she wasn't familiar with it.

She would quiz the children, who would whine while pushing and pulling at each other without really answering. It didn't take psychic powers to see where this was going. She'd eventually make her best guess as to what they wanted, and of course it was going to be completely unacceptable. There would be complaints and tears, maybe even a smacked hand as the contest of wills continued. Eventually they'd finish with no more than a couple of nibbles taken from their food, then head the mini van I could see in the parking lot with the suitcase in the luggage rack. She'd strap the little ones into their car seats, where they would soon drift off to sleep giving her an hour or so of peace as she drove.

As to where she was going, who could say? This is a military town, the home to Barksdale Air Force base. Being an Army brat myself, I know a military family when I see one. This could have been a weekend trip down to see dad, who was stationed there for a few months without family, or this may be a move to or from the base. In any case, this was obviously not a routine day for this family.

I watched the scene with the woman and her children play out pretty much as I predicted, and as the mini van disappeared down the road my heart went with them. It was such a familiar experience that I felt young again, decades away from having cancer.

Charles returned to the table holding something in a greasy wrapper as he took a seat. He washed it down with coffee as we idly chatted. I could see the sign for Regional Urology out the window, just down the road. The moment was getting closer, and harder to put out of my mind. Charles finished his breakfast and we left the restaurant.

We arrived just as the clinic was unlocking the doors. The staff showed us to the waiting room where we settled in. Somebody called my name just a few minutes later. I stood up, Charles and I shook hands and he wished me luck. As I stepped through the door, I heard somebody admonishing Charles, "Now you know you can't leave. Not even to get a cup of coffee. We've got coffee here if you want some."

I cringed. Charles doesn't deal well with people telling him what he must do or can't do. I'd forewarned him that they wanted him to stay. Unfortunately the person reiterating that now came across as bossy, even to my less sensitive ears. But my concern was unfounded. Perhaps for my benefit he was on his best behavior."Yes ma'm," he agreed, "he told me. I'll be right here."

A lady took me to the surgery prep room and showed me to a curtained cubical. "Put your clothes and valuables in here," she instructed as she handed me a plastic sack. "Then put on this gown and lay on the bed." I soon found my self again laying virtually naked under a sheet surrounded by women. This was getting to be a far too common an occurrence in my life, and not nearly as exciting as one might have imagined.

My wallet, cell phone, and other valuables were safely protected by 5 mills of polyethylene held shut by a cotton string. I'd been told to place all of that stuff in a plastic bag emblazoned with the clinic's logo. "We'll give this to your friend for safe keeping," one of the women told me as she departed with the plastic safe. "He can bring it to you after your procedure."

Another lady was soon standing by my bedside with the ever present clipboard and began going over my medical history. I assured her that I didn't have, high blood pressure, heart or lung disease, high cholesterol, or a history of cancer. No halitosis, black plague, or leprosy. She may not have actually asked about the halitosis, but then again she might have. It was a pretty through questionnaire. She then asked me about previous surgeries.

"Just knee surgery back in high school," I assured her.

"You're sure?" she asked further.

I was a little surprised and a little put off by her insistence. Did she think I was trying to keep something secret, some cosmetic surgery I didn't want to own up to? "That's all I can think of," I responded a little testily.

"Never had your tonsils or appendix out," she persisted."Maybe a hernia operation?"

Damn! Actually, I'd had two of those when I was very young. I'd had a hernia repaired before I started kindergarten, and my tonsils out during Junior High. I suddenly felt as though I'd been caught in a lie. Red faced, I admitted to the two procedures I'd forgotten.

"What hospital and who was the doctor?" she inquired.

"The tonsillectomy would have been in DeWitt City Hospital by Dr. Hester," I told her. "I can't help you much with the hernia operation. I was four or five at the time, and it would have been at some base hospital."

"What city were you in?" she asked. I could see she wasn't going to let this go easily.

"Ma'am," I said. "My dad was in the army. This happened about the time we were sent to Germany, but I can't remember whether it was before the transfer or after. I can't tell you with any certainty what country I was in, much less the city or hospital. I'm pretty sure it was on planet Earth if that helps." Giving me a baleful glare, she scribbled on the clip board for a while before finally leaving me to my own devices.

So now I lay almost naked on a bed under a single linen sheet in a room cold enough to hang beef carcasses. I could hear other patients talking to other nurses or doctors, but I don't remember any of their conversations. I don't remember if I couldn't hear them, or if nobody said anything memorable.

Not knowing how long I would have to wait, I decided to see if I could get a little sleep. I can usually drift off pretty quickly in situations like this. Even the dread of what was to come wouldn't keep me awake. I've learned to focus my mind on one of several mental places and can normally shut out nervous anticipation. The cold didn't help, but I eventually began to drift off.

It seems I'd just gone to sleep when I was awakened by the jingle of collapsing curtain rings.

The curtain was thrown open and somebody said, "Mr. Wheatley, my name is Dr ..." I didn't catch his name, but he was my anesthetist.

"I see it's been awhile since you've had any surgery," he observed as he looked over the clipboard in his hand. I'm sure it was the one the other lady had been filling out.

"No sir," I told him. "I been pretty healthy up till now."

He quizzed me again about my previous operations asking if I'd had any problems with anesthesia. I assured him I hadn't and he soon left. I had a hard time getting back to sleep, but eventually slumber did return. It was not to last long though as the rattling curtain opening awakened me again.

"It won't be long," a lady in scrubs assured me. "The doctor will be here soon and we'll get started." I lay back realizing that I'd never get to sleep again. Even if I did, I wouldn't be left along long enough to get any rest. I thought about grabbing my phone and reading something, but then I remembered it was in a plastic sack that Charles was holding for me. I had nothing to do but lay there and wait.

It probably wan't much more than ten minutes until Dr. Spinazze arrived. But ten minutes, laying mostly naked on a hard bed in a cold room with nothing to do or look at can be a very long time.

Dr Spinazze popped in for a quick visit. He went over the procedure again and asked if I had any questions. He shook my hand and told me he'd see me later. I was soon wheeled down the hall to an operating room.

THE BAD NEWS

I don't remember much about the ride home. Charles drove and I probably slept most of the way, recovering from the anesthesia. This was on a Friday and the results wouldn't be available until the following week, the last in August.

I was sporting a foley catheter after this procedure. I don't remember how long I had it. I do remember it getting blocked up and having to go to the emergency room at Wadley. My bladder began to feel full and nothing was going into the bag. I didn't wait long. As soon as I discovered I wasn't passing urine, I hot footed it over to the Wadley ER.

By the time I got there, I was starting to experience bladder spasms. The ER staff could see that I was in trouble and quickly put me in a room. I explained the situation to the male nurse who seemed to understand. "It's blocked," he told me. "I'll have to clear it by injecting some sterile water."

The thought of putting more water in my already bursting bladder didn't appeal to me, but I didn't have a better idea so I laid down and let him proceed. He filled a large syringe with sterile water, then jammed the syringe into a port in the catheter. He pushed the plunger then released it. Seconds later the relief was divine. Oh my gosh, I can't think of anything that felt better than the secession of the discomfort I'd been experiencing. I'm talking better than sex.

The young man asked where I lived and I explained that I was just a few blocks away. I could tell he was disappointed in my answer. "Well," he explained, "if you lived more than ten mile from the hospital I would be able to send a syringe and some sterile water with you so that you could clear the catheter if it got blocked again. With you this close, I'm not supposed to do that." He then set the syringe and bottle of sterile water on the counter and said he would be back in few minutes. Sharon put the syringe and water in her purse before the door was closed.

I don't remember how long I had the catheter. I don't recall being at work with it. I may have taken a day off and gone back to have it removed before returning to work. It's strange that I just can't recall.

I went back to work and tried my best to not worry about what we'd find out. Dr. Spinazze was on vacation the week following the test, so I didn't expect for him to call. But as the Labor day weekend approached, I was hoping to enjoy the three-day weekend without worrying about what I would hear Tuesday.

I called the clinic to see if I could get the results of the test. The lady transferred me to somebody who checked, then came back on the line and said, "I'm sorry, but you'll need to speak to the doctor."

That wasn't good. I'm sure she would have told me if it had been good news. I was pretty certain I could hear the bad news in her voice. If I had any doubts, she was about to dispel them. "I've got an opening Tuesday morning," she told me. "I'm setting up an appointment for you."

"I've already got an appointment scheduled for Thursday," I informed her.

"Yes sir," she acknowledged, "but I've got an opening on Tuesday, let's go ahead and get you in then." Damn! She didn't want to wait two days? This did not sound good at all. Numbly, I made the appointment then hung up. The false hope I'd been clinging too was gone.

This was the Friday before Labor day weekend and few people were around. That was good. It gave me some time to try to get myself together before I had to speak to anybody. I first thought I had it together, but soon realize I didn't. If somebody had come into my office, I'm wasn't sure I could have acted naturally.

I abandoned my office and found refuge in a secluded mezzanine area of the building where we store large bundles on pallets. I found a spot behind some boxes and let the shakes take me. I let my mind wander a little as I tried to come to grips with the likelihood that I had cancer. Even as the evidence mounted, I'd been holding onto the hope that it was something benign. This last bit of news shattered even my unbridled optimism, and I realized that I was going to have to come to terms with it.

I didn't have a prognosis yet, and maybe it wouldn't be so bad. But even as I tried to hang onto that hope, I realized that I'd been pissing blood since late June. What ever malevolence had been growing inside me had been at work since before then. That's time enough for it to have metastasized. I'm not an oncologists and didn't really understand these things, but I did know that getting to cancer early and fast is the best hope. Now I thought about the month or more I pissed away, hoping it was an infection. That was not a good decision in retrospect.

The hot acidic feeling in my stomach didn't go away, but I eventually got myself under enough control that I felt I could deal with people. I had less than an hour of work left and I was going to have to figure out what to tell Sharon.

I again grasped at the fact that I didn't really know anything. All of the hand wringing and self pity of the previous hour were based on absolutely no actual data. The only thing I knew for sure was that I had an appointment next Tuesday with my doctor to discuss the results of my tests. That was what I'd tell Sharon.

I don't remember the conversation with my wife very well, but I managed to tell her that I just didn't know anything yet and that I'd managed to get my appointment moved up to Tuesday. I think I managed to keep my dark thoughts under control enough to not damped her spirit any more than it was already.

It's odd that I don't remember the weekend. That hour Friday evening is burned so deeply into my mind that even now, six years later, it still seems like yesterday. But I have absolutely no memory of what we did that weekend. Most probably we rode the bikes somewhere with our friends.

Tuesday morning I loaded up on the bike for the now familiar ride to Shreveport. Once again I managed to talk Sharon into not going. Again, I had several reason for that. Most likely she was going to need all of the time off she could get in the coming weeks, so this was a day off with pay we could save. Then there was the idea of where I wanted to be when I gave her the news. I dreaded the thought of the hour-and-a-half long ride back home in the car after learning what I was most likely going to learn. I reasoned that I'd rather face that in the privacy of our home, with me undistracted by driving. She made me promise to call her after the appointment and before I headed home. I promised her that I would, collected a kiss and headed out.

Now-a-days, it only takes about an hour to get to Shreveport from Texarkana down I-49, but in 2011 the Interstate was still under construction. You could take it from Texarkana almost to the Louisiana State line before having to get back on Hwy. 67. I always eschewed the Interstate when on the bike, favoring the hills and curves of the older highway, even though that route added a good half-an-hour in those days.

The weather was beautiful and I tried to soak up

every moment of this motorcycle ride, likely the last I'd take to the urologists. Most probably, subsequent trips would be on I-49, as far as it went, in the car with Sharon along. Until I actually got the news, things hadn't changed yet. For the moment, I was still a biker enjoying the open road.

They didn't keep me waiting long once I reached the clinic. I'd hardly taken a seat in the waiting room when the receptionist called my name and I was ushered into an exam room with Dr. Spinazze. "Oh yeah," he said. "It's cancer and that bladder will have to come out." He forced himself to make eye contact as he delivered the news, but I think he was nervous. At least that was my impression. I think he was expecting me to react badly. Expecting bad news, my demeanor probably was not bright and chipper. I'm six-one, two-hundred-and-thirty pounds, and dressed this day in black leather riding gear. I'm a pussy cat, but I probably didn't look like somebody you wanted to get angry on that particular day.

This really wasn't news to me on an emotional level. I'd accepted that I had cancer last Friday. Today was just learning how bad it was, so I don't think I really reacted. I seem to show less emotion when I'm scared. I try to handle the fear with logic, by trying to understand the threat as much as possible and figure out how to deal with it. "So we're looking at surgery to remove the cancer?" I asked the doc.

He seemed surprised at my mild reaction but quickly recovered and got back to business. "We'll have to remove the entire bladder," he clarified, and I felt the first shock of the visit so far. Like I said, I tend to get quiet when frightened and I was very quiet at this news. As the doctor began to layout the situation to me, I didn't react and I suspect he thought I wasn't grasping what he was telling me. He kept asking me if I understood. I did, and it scared me enough that I just listened even more quietly. It was a good news, bad news situation.

I wasn't going to have to go through chemotherapy or radiation treatment, so I was going to be spared the hair loss and nausea that comes with that. The bad news was that the reason I wouldn't have to endure those treatments was because the particular cancer I had laughed that shit off the way a pitbull would laugh off a yorkie. Those treatments offered so little potential of doing anything good that the doctor wouldn't subject me to the side effects. Our only hope was to surgically remove the cancer. If it was confined to my bladder, then I had a good chance. If it had spread further, the chances were not so good. I'm pretty sure plan B was to send me home with the number of a local Hospice.

Because we only had one shot at this, the doctor wasn't willing to take a chance of only removing the tumor. The whole bladder was going to have to come out. This is where Dr. Spinazze and I would part company. "I'm too old to do that kind of surgery any more," he told me. "I've spoken with a colleague who will take the case. He will talk with you after his last appointment today if you want to wait."

It was a little after four in the afternoon by now and Dr. Spinazze thought I'd be able to meet with Dr. Henderson in about an hour. I agreed and thanked him. He left me in the exam room to wait on my new surgeon.

I suspected this whole living without a bladder thing was going to prove inconvenient. The Internet is a wonderful thing. I had, in my pocket, a marvelous device that allowed me access to almost the sum total of human knowledge. I used it now to try and understand as much as I could about what I was facing. I learned that removing the bladder is called a radical cystectomy. The information available to me at the time described a procedures where the ureters, that run from my kidneys to my bladder, would be replaced by an ileal conduit running to a structure called a stoma they would construct on my abdomen. Urine would flow from here into an ostomy bag that I would wear on my side.

Wow, it was getting hard to see the screen on my phone. I don't remember if it was because my hands were shaking or my eyes just couldn't look at what I was seeing. I tried to imagine what life was going to be like after the surgery. How intrusive was the ostomy bag going to be? Would I still be able to ride the motorcycle? Would I be able to be intimate with my wife?

I'm sure I suffered some emotional overload during that hour as I waited and read, but it was a good thing. I was absorbing the shock by the time

Dr. Henderson came into the room I was over the worst of it and knew enough to ask some pertinent questions. I went right to the worst part first. "Will I have a stoma?" I asked.

"Well that is one option," the doctor answered, "but I'm recommending a different solution. I suggest we go with a neobladder."

Because I was still fairly young, fifty-five at the time, and in otherwise good health, I was eligible for this option. The doctor would remove my cancerous bladder, prostate, and seminal vesicle, then replace the natural bladder with a neobladder made from a section of my small intestine. Given time, I had every reasonable expectation of resuming a fairly normal life.

The doctor kept watching me as he explained the procedure. He must have been expecting to see concern or maybe even fear at the prospect he was laying out. I was suddenly learning that I was escaping the horrors I'd been expecting the last hour. Hell, I was almost giddy.

He didn't want to wait and told me he was going to schedule the surgery as soon as he could find a hospital with an available operating room. He thought it would likely be in less than a week. This surprised me and reminded me that I still wasn't out of the woods. The almost normal life I was still swooning over would not be possible if the cancer had spread past my bladder. I was still possibly under a death sentence. But that had always been the worst case scenario. Now at least the best case was so much better than I had hoped.

He kept asking if I understood and eventually asked if I wanted to set up another appointment so that I could bring my wife and we could discuss it some more. It was obvious that my muted reaction was giving him the impression that I wasn't grasping the seriousness of the situation, or maybe that I just didn't understand what was happening. "Are you going to tell me anything then that you haven't told me now?" I asked.

He seemed surprised by my question as he said, "No. I just want to be sure you don't have any questions."

"I think you've explained things pretty thoroughly," I told him. "I think I can explain it to my wife. Let's just get this over with." He warned me that I might get calls from more than one hospital as he was checking with several to see which one would have the first opening. We shook hands and I was soon standing in the parking lot contemplating the phone call I was about to make.

I could hear the concern in her voice when Mrs. Sharon answered the phone. "It's after five," she admonished. "I thought maybe you'd forgot to call." Now she was protecting me, trying to not worry me with her fear. What she really thought was that I had bad news and was just going to wait until I got home to break it to her. It was a reasonable assumption on her part as I had considered doing just exactly that. I might have done that if there hadn't been a positive aspect to focus on.

I saw no reason to drag this out, so I lead off

with the bad news. "It's cancer," I said, "but," I quickly added, "the doctor thinks he can remove it and things sound better than I expected. I'll possibly be back to normal in a few months." I begged off further explanations saying it was a bit complex and that I'd go over all of it with her when I got home. I closed the connection with the reminder that after surgery I might well be completely cured. I told her I loved her and asked her to not worry, then gassed up and headed for home.

The ride home was introspective. I'd primarily been focusing on what we were doing to beat this since the diagnosis. But underlaying that hope was the very real possibility that this thing had already escaped my bladder. If that were the case, then I was a dead man walking. I decided that now, while I still had the potential of hope to retreat to, was the time to take the first mental steps down that path. I was going to try and feel out this possibility, to partially immunize my self to the fear from the safety of a place where I still had hope.

I would be spared having to make decisions about treatment, whether or not to subject myself to chemo and radiation in the hopes of buying time. With my cancer, that wasn't an option. I just had to figure out how I was going to handle the end if it came to that. I knew that I was not going to spend my last days, helpless and in pain, possibly begging for somebody to end my suffering, knowing that they wouldn't, couldn't. If leaving this world was inevitable, then I do it on my own terms.

That decision made, the next one was how I'd go

about it. Eating a gun would be the easiest for me, but that would leave a mess and be hard on Mrs. Sharon. I decided it would be best if it wasn't clearly a suicide. I'd wait as long as possible, but before I became helpless, I'd take one last motorcycle ride.

The Talimena scenic drive is a beautiful stretch of road that runs the crest of Rich Mountain from Mena Arkansas to Talihina Oklahoma. I would just pick the right curve and see where the outside of the envelope was. I could take it faster and faster until I discovered the limit of man and machine to hold the road. In a way, it almost wouldn't have been suicide. It's not like I'd have just ridden over the edge, I would have truly been trying to hold it, but been unable because of taking the curve too fast. I'm sure those who knew me would suspect it was intentional, but at least I'd be offering my loved ones the chance to accept the version they could best live with.

I'd have to pick a spot where there was no hope of survival. I didn't want to just mess myself up real bad and wind in a hospital. No, I'd have to make sure that where the accident happened, it was going to be fatal.

I saw several downsides to this plan. For one thing, I was going to destroy a beautiful motorcycle that otherwise could have gone to my son. I felt bad about that, but was willing to accept the selfishness of it to spare them, and me, something far worse. Also, even in the best case scenario, there would be a few seconds of fear as I flew helplessly into the abyss. Hopefully I'd hit hard enough to die instantly, but there was always the possibility of a painful death.

The worst part of it would be that long ride from Texarkana to Mena, knowing that I would never see Sharon again. That last kiss promising to see her tonight, knowing I wouldn't.

I considered those things on that long lonely ride home from the clinic. Hopefully these were morbid musings that would never come to be. For the moment, I still had a fighting chance of surviving this thing, and it was time to return my focus to that.

The hospital

Sharon listened much more stoically than I anticipated. I suspect that, like me, she had been battling her own fear and that the news I was giving her now, bad as it was, wasn't as bad as what she had feared. I suppose it's also possible that I heavily emphasized the positive and down played the negative aspects. I kept mentioning that in a few months I could be cancer free and back to normal.

Dr. Henderson was right in that I got a call from a couple of hospitals to set up pre-admission interviews. I called the clinic to see which one they wanted me to use and got an appointment for the interview. They told me what all to bring with me, which included insurance papers, lists of medication I was taking, and a thousand dollars.

Well crap, here we go again. Having cancer is bad enough, but the financial strain on top of that was horrible. I'm not going to relive that hideous time, but we were able to come up with the money by cashing in a life insurance policy. We were spared having to sell some of the land Sharon owned back in Arkansas County. We wound up borrowing the thousand from our son until the check from the life insurance came.

I was told that I'd be off work for six to eight weeks. Fortunately, I had eight weeks of paid time built up in sick leave and vacation, so at least pay checks would keep coming.

I hadn't made an announcement at work yet though I had told the few people who legitimately needed to know. Three people in particular were going to have to cover for me and they deserved to have as much warning as I could give them to prepare. I didn't want the word to get out yet to anybody else. Once those words leave your mouth, they can't be unsaid. You're talking to somebody and you're normal. Then you say those words and suddenly things are different and you can't go back. I discovered that I desperately wanted to hold onto the normal as long as I could.

I drafted a memo and presented at the next department head meeting. I asked the other department heads to wait until the day I left, Friday, to pass out the memos. Of course, somebody didn't listen and distributed it right after the meeting on Tuesday morning. I'll include he text of the memo below. I've removed the name of employees mentioned by name:

To: My Gazette Family

From: Guy Wheatley

Date: September 21, 2011

Re: Extended Leave

After this Friday, September 23, I will be taking an extended leave. Possibly as long as 6 to 8 weeks. I will be undergoing treatment for bladder cancer in Shreveport. I should be able to leave the hospital in 7 to 10 days, but will be convalescing for an extended time. The good news is that after the surgery, the cancer will be gone. Hopefully I can return to work in less than 2 months and be back to almost completely normal within a year.

During my absence, technical issues should be addressed to XXX XXXXXXX's capable hands. XXXX XXXXX with the help of XXXXX XXXXX will manage pre-press production. XXXX XXXXX has generously volunteered to take over production items during the day, such as eye jackets, and TC News.

Up until this point, I've told only those people that necessity required. People who needed time to prepare to assume new responsibilities during my absence. Please do not be offended by this decision on my part. It in no way reflects negatively on my opinion of any of my friends and coworkers. It was simply a result of my desire to keep my life as normal as possible for as long as possible.

Facing this part of my life, I am so grateful to be a member of the Texarkana Gazette family. I've worked for other companies and have watched the companies my wife worked for. I have never experienced any other place that so warmly embraces a member in need. I want to express a heartfelt thanks to each and everyone of you who have made this such a wonderful place to live and work. From the porters, always ready with a joke or friendly jibe, to Mr. Hussman, who provided the environment in which this wonderful culture has developed, thank you.

Your warm thoughts and prayers are welcome. I will try to keep you informed as to my progress. I already miss you guys and look forward to returning to the fold.

With the early distribution of the memo came the dreaded goodbyes and well wishing from coworkers. Don't get me wrong, I appreciated their sincere concern and well wishes. But after some number of times of adopting the long suffering expression as I thanked them, it began to feel artificial on my part. I was really hoping my last few days at work before the surgery would just be normal, ordinary days.

The lucky facility that would host my operation turned out to be Christus Schumpert Highland on Bert Kouns highway. Mrs. Sharon's neurology doctor is just a few blocks north on Youree drive and I'm familiar with this area. I was a little disappointed at first.

Shreveport has several hospitals situated in towering buildings and I suppose I assumed I'd be in one of those. In my mind, I was equating the hight of the building with the technical prowess of the institution. Christus Schumpert Highland is out on the industrial loop and the tallest build in the complex is three stories. Much of it is single story and I know that in my mind I was equating it to some of the rural, county hospitals I've been to.

Now I don't want to dog on these rural hospitals, because they fill an important niche. But the simple truth of the matter is that most of these places are not on the cutting edge of medicine and can only handle rather routine procedures. Growing up in the country we often equated the seriousness of a person's illness by where their doctor sent them. If it was DeWitt City Hospital, then it wasn't a big deal, something routine like having a baby or getting your tonsils out. If things got a tad more serious, they might send you on to Stuttgart or Pine Bluff. This was usually because you needed a specialists. Lord help you if they'd packed your carcass off to Little Rock. Hell, we'd just about start planning your funeral if you were that bad off.

This was the mindset with which I eyed the low laying buildings at Christus Schumpert Highland. Looking back now, I can see the many flaws in that "logic." I've never had better care, or better nurses and given the choice, I don't think I'd go anywhere else were I to again need surgery.

Me being me, I had to learn as much as I could about the coming operation. Like I said earlier, the Internet is a wonderful thing. With more time, more information to start with, and a laptop instead of a smart phone, I had access to much more online material. I couldn't find video of a neobladder reconstruction, but I eventually I eventually found one of a radical cystectomy. That was intense to watch, especially knowing that I was soon to under go a similar procedure. But I did feel better now that I had a pretty good understanding of what was going to happen to me.

Saturday was my last day as a regular person. Sunday I'd have to stop eating and start using the Fleet enemas. Yeah buddy. Sometime when you're just killing time, stop by the pharmacy and check out the instructions on the Fleet enema box. Shouldn't be a problem if you're a contortionists or into yoga.

Because the doc was going to cut out a segment of my small intestine, I had to be especially emptied out, so this wasn't a one time procedure. This was even more intense than prepping for a colonoscopy. I don't remember the details, but I'm pretty sure I had to stop eating twenty-four hours before time and took at least a couple of enemas. I don't remember drinking the nasty stuff that gave you the runs, but that must surely have been part of the program.

Then I started trying to get my heard around what was going to happen. In addition to my bladder, I was about to lose my prostate and seminal vesicle. I would no longer produce semen. That realization had a greater psychological impact on me than I expected. I was fifty-five and had no intention of having anymore children. It's possible that my aged sperm wasn't even viable anymore, but there was still the possibility. In a few hours, that was going to be forever gone, and the pending loss was more profound than I anticipated. I was losing something that was more precious to me than I realized.

Brandon, our son, had come home on Friday and would accompany us to Shreveport Monday morning. My daughter, her husband and the grandkids were flying into Shreveport and had a hotel room. They would meet us at the hospital. I set out a couple of extra litter pans for the cats and made sure they had enough food and water for several days. Brandon would stop by and check on them in a couple of days on his way back to Fort Worth. We had just gotten a yorkie puppy a week before. He was staying with Charles and Brenda. The bigger dogs would stay in the back yard with enough dry food to last until we got back. Our next door neighbor would check on them. Brandon would check on them also as he came through town.

I don't remember what time the surgery was scheduled for, but I know it was in the morning. I think about eight or so. It would take five hours or more, so everybody had hauled in the books, laptops, and tablets, you see in waiting rooms now days. I, of course, would sleep through it all.

I don't recall waiting very long, but then it's not like I was anxious to get started either. Soon, however, a nurse came to get me and take me for preparation. I hugged everybody and we all assured each other everything was going to be fine and we'd see each other soon. The nurse directed my family to a different waiting room as she escorted me to the prep area.

In no time, I was once again laying naked, under a sheet, surrounded by women. The experience still wasn't growing on me.

After The Surgery

I was once again interrogated by a lady holding a clipboard. I remembered about the tonsillectomy and hernia operations this time, though I still didn't know what continent I was on when the hernia was repaired.

Dr. Henderson arrived accompanied by a body guard. This guy was massive and ripped. I mean he could have been the Incredible Hulk if he was just green and maybe a bit smaller. He was wearing scrubs and began to ask me questions about allergies to medication. I finally realized that this wasn't a body guard after all, he was the anesthetists.

I think Dr. Henderson asked if I had any questions, and I probably said I didn't. At some point we shook hands and he told me he'd see me after the surgery.

A short time later a couple of people wheeled me to the operating room and helped me onto the operating table. You hear of people who just don't wake up from anesthesia, but that was rare. I knew that the odds were overwhelmingly in my favor, still I couldn't get it out of my mind that there was a chance I'd never wake up.

My memory starts getting fuzzy here. I know I was awake when the Hulk came in to put me to sleep, but I don't really remember it. Then at some point I was in a different room, surrounded by people. I think Sharon was there. I was in a hospital bed and as I began to come around I was surprised at the number of people wearing scrubs surrounding me.

As I began to come more fully awake, somebody ran off most of the people in scrubs. The one who stayed smiled at me sheepishly and said, "I'm sorry, but we've never seen somebody who had as many procedures at one time. They just wanted to see you." Wow, I was a celebrity.

At some point, over the next few days, I came to understand the magnitude of what Dr. Henderson had done. I basically had five surgeries at the same time. There was the removal of my bladder of course, but then there was also a bowel resection once they harvested the section of small intestine they made my new bladder from. Then there was the marvel of making a new bladder, the removal of my prostate, and the final pièce de résistance was the temporary diversion of urine to an ostomy bag using an ileal conduit from my kidneys to a hole in my side. A coupe of plastic tubes were sticking out of a hole in my side and I had an ostomy bag glued over them that the urine filled with a steady drip from my kidneys. This was a temporary measure to give my new, store bought, bladder time to heal before using it.

The room I was in was small and only held my bed, but I soon came to understand it was still a recovery room, not the hospital room I would eventually be assigned. The young man in scrubs told us that according to the rules I could only have one visitor with me and then for only a few minutes. But he said that as long as nobody called him on it, he'd let Donya and Brandon stay with us as well. Donya's husband and the grandkids eventually joined us and nobody ever squawked.

I wasn't in pain, but I itched to high heaven. I had compression cuffs on my legs and I couldn't get to my legs to scratch. I started looking around the room for something I could use to stick in the cuffs and scratch with. Donya volunteered to check the gift shop to see if they had something I could use. The only thing she found was a bright pink ruler.

Dr. Henderson stoped by just as Donya arrived back in my room with the ruler. He got a funny look on his face when she handed it to me and said, "Dad, I got you this at the gift shop." He was probably even more confused with my obvious glee at the gift. Then he laughed harder than I'd ever heard him laugh before when I shoved it down the leg cuffs and began to vigorously relieve the itching.

Morphine!

I've heard people sing it's high praises after surgery. It didn't work out that way for me. Before I was taken to my regular room, the Hulk came in and explained the box on the pole. A box containing morphine was fixed to a pole and attached to me. It delivered a small dose at a steady rate, but if I were in pain, I could press a button and get a larger dose. There was a limit to how much of the happy juice I could get the box to dispense, but it was supposed to be a high enough dose to help with pain.

The only real problem was that I wasn't in pain. What's more, I soon came to find out that the incessant itching I was experiencing was likely due to the morphine. Nurses would come in, check the box and see that I hadn't pressed the magic button. They would assume I was unaware of it and explain its function. Of course they would want to demonstrate by pressing it. Fortunately, I had a nifty pink ruler to help dissuade such demonstrations. Word soon got around the ward that if you didn't want your knuckles rapped, to keep you fingers off of that damn button.

The Incredible Hulk came by the next day to check on me. I learned that in addition to administering the anesthesia, he was in charge of my pain management. He noticed that I hadn't been using the magic button and like everybody else assumed that I was unaware of it. The ruler stayed at my side as he reached toward it to demonstrate its use. They removed my bladder, not my brain.

I did manage to stop him from pressing it with a heart felt plea. I explained that I simply wasn't in pain and that the itching the drug was likely causing was far more uncomfortable that any post surgical discomfort it was supposed to relieve. He looked at me as though I'd been speaking Swahili. Eventually his mind was able to translate the sounds I was making to the communication that I did not want the drug. I think he was a bit insulted. "Well if you're not going to use it, we might as well unhook it," he said somewhat testily.

I'd been fantasizing about getting that damn thing off of me since I woke up. Even without pressing the button, it was delivering a minimal dose that kept me clawing at my hide. Now though, at the prospect of having it removed, I suddenly felt some hesitation. I hadn't been in pain, but I knew that the button was right there if things ever got bad enough to endure the itching. Now that option was about to be removed. I thought about it for a few seconds, then said, "I guess I can take a pill if I start hurting, right?" The Hulk allowed that I was correct, so I agreed to have the itch box removed.

Because we were so desperate to get the procedure going, I was checked in to the hospital in an expeditious manor. It happened so quickly that some of the support services weren't assigned. Among those was physical therapy. Modern medical philosophy seems to be stick a new heart into your chest Tuesday, then have you run a marathon Wednesday. Somehow, my PT guy didn't get by until Wednesday, three days after my surgery.

I'd been laying flat on my back for three days. I was bound by compression cuffs on my legs that the amount of money I could command as a bribe was insufficient to have removed. But the biggest incentive to lay still and not cause problems was the uncertain incision in my belly. It seemed to me that an unfortunate cough or sneeze would spill my innards out onto my lap.

Dr. Henderson had been by several times and I came to understand that my intestines were not moving. Your Intestines are supposed to squirm around inside of you like a ball of procreating snakes as they work food through them. The trauma of having a section cut out of it and being sewed back together had paralyzed mine. I would be unable to eat anything until I could get my innards moving again. One of the things that would help that happen would be walking. Hence, my consternation about the Physical Therapy guy not showing for three days.

He finally arrived Wednesday afternoon and I was going to try and stand for the first time since Monday morning. The idea was I'd try to walk to the door and back. He strapped me up in some sort of BDSM harness that he would use to support me if I was unable to stand on my own. This guy was a buck fifty at most soaking wet. As I mentioned earlier, I tip the scales at two-thirty. Well maybe two-twenty by now. Make that two-fifteen. Still, bondage equipment or not, I didn't have a lot of faith this little fellow could keep me on my feet if my lights went out.

The little guy kept cautioning me to go easy. He even suggested that we just have me sit on the edge of the bed on this first attempt. I wasn't having any of that. I was going for a walk down the hallway. I had more trouble than I expected just sitting up, but

I managed to make it to the side of the bed. I swung my legs over and things went dark for a second. The PT guy held my shoulders and admonished me to just take it easy for a minute.

The world again appeared out of the fog and I was able to sit on the side of the bed without assistance. I sat there for a while and the PT guy suggested that this was enough for our first attempt. No way. I had a date with the hallway and I was going to keep it. I slid carefully off the edge of the bed and allowed my feet to take my full weight.

I'm not sure what happened next. The diminutive PT guy was stouter than he looked. I either stepped or fell forward a couple of steps because when I started to come back to myself, he was actually supporting me with the bondage harness and managed to haul my limp tuckus back to the bed. He got me seated and after I sat there a while, I was able to think again. "Are you ready to lay down?" he asked.

"Yeah," I agreed.

Pre-surgery, I had seven holes leading to my anatomical interior. One mouth, two ears, two nostrils, one rectum, and one urethra. Awakening from surgery I found that I was a much more assessable organism. In addition to the seven orifices I came into the world with, I now had a hole in my side for the ileal conduit, two drain tubes, and a huge needle in a vein in the back of my hand for easy delivery of the things they thought it would be a good idea to inject into my body.

I mentioned the pole the itch box was attached

to, but there were other devices on it as well. Wires ran from sensor pads glued to my body back to devices on the pole that had various lights, displays, and buttons. That damn thing looked like some sort of dystopian Christmas tree. It also held bags of normal saline and a tube ran from it to the vein in the back of my hand. The urine bag from my catheter also had a home on the pole. Where I went, the pole went.

My physical therapists came back the next day and I managed to make it to the door. I did actually take a step into the hall, but he didn't have to chide me to get me to head back to the bed. As my strength increased over the next few days, I was able to walk further and further. By Friday I was on my own and able to accomplish what I called, "making the block." I'd step into the hall, then head one direction or the other down to the next hall. I'd turn down the new hallway to the next intersection and make another ninety degree turn. This would take me back to the passage my room was on.

As I mentioned earlier, where I went the pole went. On my first couple of excursions, I was glad to have it. It was the only thing that kept me on my feet several times. But as I got better and no longer needed it for support, it became nothing more than a nuisance. Even trips to the bathroom for a much anticipated and hoped for bowel movement meant dragging the pole with me.

Surgery and an extended stay in the hospital will certainly change your priorities. My whole being was now focus on walking as far as the door to my room, and making a poo-poo. The last thing other than water I'd had by mouth was Saturday bight. By Thursday, I was ready for some food, but I couldn't eat until my intestines began moving again. We'd know this blessed event had occurred when I had a bowel movement, hence my intense interest in making a poo-poo. I'd been dragging the pole to the bathroom for a couple of days now in the hopes of accomplishing this goal. Some time Thursday, I managed something close enough that Dr. Henderson said he might allow me to try something solid for breakfast Friday morning.

Mrs. Sharon ran to the cafeteria bright and early and bought a sausage, cheese, and egg biscuit. We then waited anxiously for Dr. Henderson to come in and give me the final blessing for a solid breakfast. He came in and listened to my stomach with his stethoscope, then gave us the thumbs up. I was go for sausage.

I thought I'd wolf the thing down in one bite. I nibbled some crumbs from the biscuit. It turns out that if you don't put anything into your stomach for five days, it shrinks. It took me a couple of hours, but with determination, I conquered the breakfast sandwich. I enjoyed what I would have previously considered very small meals for lunch, dinner, and breakfast Saturday morning.

The kids all left by Tuesday evening and Mrs. Sharon had not left my side since then. Though my room was a double occupancy, I was the only patient assigned to it, and the hospital staff was kind enough to offer the other bed for Sharon. Now, on

Saturday morning she was needing a few supplies, and possibly a short break from the hospital. I assured her that I would be just fine on my own for a couple of hours while she did some shopping. Besides, I had a hospital full of attentive nurses. So shortly after breakfast, still with some trepidation, she gave me a kiss and headed out.

She probably hadn't gotten to the parking lot when I realized that I was about to toss my cookies. With the leg cuffs on, there was no way I could get out of bed on my own, and there was nothing within reach that I could use. The call button was intergraded with the television remote that Sharon had been using, and was out of reach on the other bed.

I tried to reach the cuffs to remove them, but that was not going to happen. My innards were barely held inside of me by the staples closing the incision. The surgeon had to cut through my abdominal muscles to reach the broken bits he repaired and they were not healed enough yet for me to do the sit up required to reach the cuffs on my own. I was trapped on my back like a tortoise. It looked as though I was about to toss everything I'd eaten since yesterday morning right onto those afore mentioned staples. That was not a pleasant prospect.

I could see a kidney shaped pan setting on a side table, just out of my reach. My only hope was to get somebody in the hall to come in and give it to me. I tried to call for help, but I could taste bile at the back of my throat and feel the contents of my stomach floating just below where my tonsils would be if I still had them. My tongue was curled in an attempt to present a barricade to the escaping breakfast sausage and it's companions, so I couldn't form an L sound. "Hep! Hep!" was all I could weakly say. Between weakened abdominal muscles and fear of pressure releasing the acidic flood at the back of my throat, I wasn't making much sound.

Fortunately a lady passing in the hall did hear me. She poked her head thorough my door and her eyes went wide. I'm not sure what frightened her so badly, whether she was picking up on my panic, or whether I just looked that bad. She pulled back out of the door to make a hasty get-a-way, but my pitiful "Hep!" must have called her back. She poked her head back around the corner and I desperately pointed to the pan. "Pan! Pan!" was all I could get out as I desperately jabbed my finger at it.

Her eyes were wide as she followed my gesture. She took a few timid steps into my room, far enough to be able to reach the pan. She then leaned toward my bed, staying as far away as possible from me as she tossed to pan toward me. Was I glowing green? Did she think I was radioactive?

Her aim was good enough that the pan hit the over-the-bed table and bounced onto the bed. I grabbed it and released the meals I'd barely been holding captive. The lady was out the door before the food was out of my mouth. I'm not sure exactly what she feared I might disgorge. Maybe she'd seen the movie "Alien," recently. I never saw her again, but I was certainly grateful for her brief, if reluctant, appearance.

LEAVING THE HOSPITAL

I soon began to chart my progress by the number of connections to the pole that were removed. I don't remember the sequence the connections were severed. I know that the itch box was the first thing to go. I think that the monitors were next. Eventually, once I was able to take food and water by mouth, we were able to dispense with the normal saline drip. I could hang the urine bag the catheter drained into and the ostomy bag from hooks on the bed while I was laying in it. I would wear them with straps and harnesses when ambulatory.

I was thrilled once that last connection was gone. For what ever reason, they left the pole right where it had held station at the side of my bed, but it was now dark and I knew that my next excursion would be without it. I drifted off to sleep, happy in my new found independence.

Sometime later I awakened and realized I needed to go to the bathroom. I grabbed the pole and shoved it in front of me as I crossed the room. I did the pirouette at the bathroom door and pulled the pole as far into the bathroom as its wide base would allow so that I could reach the toilet. Once seated, I began the routine check to be sure none of the wires and tubes would get tangled in my feet. Then I started laughing. I laughed so hard I began to be concerned about the staples holding my innards safely inside of me.

"Sharon," I called.

"What?" she asked with concern in her voice as she rushed to the bathroom door.

"Look what I've done," I said, pointing at the pole. She examined the pole, trying to see what was wrong or different about it. She looked at me with a questioning expression. "I'm not hooked to it any more," I said. I'd hauled that thing around with me so long it had become second nature. I'd sleepily hauled it with me without realizing that I was now free of it.

Mrs. Sharon also began to laugh. It had been a long times since I'd hear that musical sound.

— — —

I was getting stronger, and simply making the block wasn't enough any more. I noticed a sign pointing to a chapel and I felt an overwhelming urge to go there. I followed the hall I thought lead to the chapel, but was unable to locate it. It was important to me to find this place, but my strength was fading and I reluctantly turned back toward my room. Turning down the hall in which the door to my room was located, I finally noticed that the chapel was in a converted hospital room, just a few doors down from mine. I'd missed it because I was expecting something larger. I didn't understand the relief when I found it.

I quietly entered and discovered an alter at the far end. Small pews lined both sides with an isle from the door to the alter. I was alone. No. That's not right. I was the only human visible in the room. I soon understood that I was not alone.

I'm very spiritual, but I'm not superstitious. The laws of physics explains how the universe works and the constraints on what can happen. I'm extremely skeptical of supposed miracles. Keep in mind that the laws of physics were not set in place by some scientist. The speed of light is set at roughly 186,000 miles per second. That value wasn't set by some scientist. It is generally accepted that a scientist named Olaus Roemer first measured the speed of light, be he didn't set the value. The value was set by the creator of the universe. In my world view, that is God of Abraham, my God. So when some supposed miracle worker violates, the laws of physics, he is actually violating laws that God has set in place. I have grave doubt that actually happen often, if at all. I don't think God has to back up ten and punt because of the unintended consequences of one of his laws. I don't need miracles to know God.

But God has touched me very profoundly several times in my life, and this was to be the most wonderful so far. As I stood there, I had the powerful feeling that some somebody standing behind me, with his hand on my shoulder. The sensation was overwhelming and I began to sob uncontrollably. I was completely taken in some strong emotion, though I'm not certain what that emotion was. I could feel God assuring me that it was OK. Not that I was going to beat the cancer or make a full recovery. That's not what he meant by OK. What ever happened, he would be with me and I would be OK.

I didn't want the moment to end. I wanted to stay there forever. But as world shattering as this was to me, it was still just a pat on the shoulder, a kiss on the forehead, not a promise of an outcome.

I hung onto that memory for weeks. I tried to relive it and even tried to turn it into some epiphanic moment. But that's not what it was. It was a much needed, and divinely profound pat on the back reminding me that he loved me and would be with me through what ever came next.

— — —

Sunday evening Dr.Henderson came by and asked if I'd like to go home in the morning. I told him that if my wife wasn't in the room, I'd kiss him. He laughed, looked at Sharon and said, "Well I'm certainly glad you're here."

Monday morning became Monday afternoon, but I eventually found myself in a wheel chair, being pushed toward the front entrance of the hospital. Sharon brought the cavalier around and with ample assistance from Sharon and nurses, I managed to get into the passenger seat. Brandon called as we were making the loop around Shreveport. Distracted, I pointed Mrs. Sharon to the wrong exit. We were now on I-20 west, heading for Dallas rather than Texarkana.

I don't know why, whether it was the weakness, residual effect of the drugs, or the simple fact that even the simplest of things required an enormous amount of effort and determination. But my temper was now on an extremely short fuse and I would snap at Sharon more than I care to remember over the next couple of weeks. This was the first of those occasions.

We eventually got back on the right track home, but by now Sharon was upset. We hit a couple of rough spots in the road pretty hard and I was truly afraid of pulling my incision apart. I still couldn't contract my stomach muscles to hold my intestines in place and every jolt really felt like I was about to spill my innards into the floorboard. Looking back, it would have served me right. I got pretty snippy several times with the woman who had stood by me thorough this and all I've thrown at her during our marriage. It wasn't my finest hour.

We finally got home with my insides still inside of me. Sharon helped me into the house and settled me on the couch. I needed help to even get to my feet and was under strict orders to not carry anything, so that left it to Sharon to do everything else. I just sat on the couch watching TV, still using my hands to delicately hold in my innards at every deep breath or cough as Sharon spent the rest of the evening hauling in stuff from the car getting supper and cleaning up what messes the cats had left.

We'd left the cats with sufficient litter pans, food and water to hold out for the seven to ten days we'd expected to be gone. Brandon had come by on his way home on Tuesday to check on them. He must not have done a head count. One of them had managed to dart unseen through the door to our bedroom, which we closed to keep off limits, as we left.

This rotund ball of gray stripped fur goes by the ridiculous nom de plume Skinny Minnie. Though the name fit when she came to us, it has been many years since she could fit in her prom dress. I'd taken to calling her Fatty Patty, however Mrs Sharon nixed that name. So even as we watch her waddle down the hall, as wide or tall as she is long, we still call her Skinny Minnie. It's amazing how she can get that much fat moving so fast so quickly, but she can. And of course she picked the worst possible time to do it, dashing unseen through a door that would remain closed for the next seven days.

As we opened the bedroom door that night, headed for blessed slumber, a much more svelte Skinny Minnie zipped between our legs in a mad dash to the feeder and water dish. It became quickly obvious that we would not be sleeping in our bed this night.

Settling down in the guest bedroom, I lay in bed with the Yorkie puppy Charles and Brenda had returned a few hours earlier. We had a rug topped with towels on the bed, that was his bed. Sharon finished her chores and came to bed. Leaving her and the Yorkie, I went to the bathroom to start swapping and cleaning the various bags and tubes that would be my constant companions for the next four or five weeks. Just as I was finishing up, I heard a distressed, 'Oh no! BINKY!" I guess there was just too much change and too much excitement for that little bladder. Sharon had stepped out of bed for just a second to grab another blanket. Binky stepped off his bed for some other business. On to the second guest bedroom, and our third bed for the night. Thus passed our first evening home.

— — —

I continued to go outside often and began walking up and down the side walk. I could make it to the end of the block by the end of the second day. Sharon would stay home another couple of days and kept an eagle eye on me, admonishing me to not go too far. She knows me too well. I've always been a little too big for my britches and often pushed myself beyond my limits. She knew that I was anxious to regain my strength and concerned that I'd walk too far, then be unable to get back home.

The sidewalk in front of the house was becoming very familiar to me and boring. It occurred to me that walking it four times, would be the equivalent to walking around the block, so after proving my stamina equal to that, I decided to see some new pavement on my next excursion. At the end of the block, I made a right and headed off down the sidewalk toward the next intersection. I still felt pretty good by the time I got there and reasoned that I was all ready almost half way around the block. It was only a little further if I kept going as compared to turning back, so I plowed ahead.

By the time I got to the next street I was slowing considerably, but by now it really was shorter to continue on rather than retrace my steps. It felt like two, or maybe three blocks up to that next intersection. I was winded by the time I approached the last turn onto my street. I could hear Sharon calling for me, but didn't have the breath left to holler back. As I made the corner our next door neighbor saw me and called to Sharon, "Here he is."

I waved feebly as I slowly hobbled up the sidewalk toward home. I almost turned and made a run for it when I saw the look Mrs. Sharon was giving me. I would have if I'd had the strength. She called back the neighbors that had fanned out looking for me.

By the next day I was able to convince Mrs. Sharon to go back to work. I was able to get around the house pretty well. My plans were to stay on the couch, but if I needed to run to the bathroom or kitchen I was now strong enough to do it. She needed to do something beside look after me, and frankly, I needed to start doing for myself again. She still had some paid leave available, but I convinced her that I would be all right and she might as well save the time for later.

I hate being stuck in front of the television during the day. There just isn't enough stuff to keep my interest all day. I'd planned to use the time I'd have convalescing to write. I don't really remember how I filled the days, but it wasn't writing. I did a little writing, but not as much as I thought I would. I think I pretty much slept and stayed on the Internet.

THE FIRST EXCURSIONS

By the next weekend I was feeling much stronger. More salient was that I was going stir crazy. I had to get out of the house for a while. I had another consideration beside my weakened condition. In addition to the ostomy bag for the ileal conduit, I also still had the foley catheter. I was able to wear the bag from the catheter low on my leg, just above the ankle with a tube running down my leg. Most of the urine my body produced in those days exited through the ileal conduit and was therefore collected in the ostomy bag attached to my side. That's inconvienetiely high to carry that much liquid. Fortunately the bag had a port at the bottom and I was able to run a tube from it to the lower bag strapped just above my ankle. I had more plumbing on me than a sauna.

I was able to keep the tubes and bags out of sight under clothing that was now loose after my hospital stay. I didn't look like a cyborg, but it was still hard to move with all of that stuff attached to me. The most restricting factor was the catheter. When seepage leaked around the tube, it slid easily in its passage and wasn't particularly uncomfortable. On those occasions when the foley bulb sealed against the opening from by bladder and my urethra stayed dry, the tube would stick and pull painfully as it moved with my body. I preferred dealing with the urine soaked mucus discharge over the sticking.

My first trip away from the house was with Mrs. Sharon to Walmart. I hobbled into the store and selected one of the riding carts they provide. That thing was slower than a molasses water fall. I was sitting too low to see over the crowd nor could I reach anything without standing up. I'm entirely too type A to put up with that thing and quickly abandoned it. The catheter wasn't sticking at the moment so I was fairly ambulatory. A shopping cart made a handy walker and I used it to complete my business.

For all of the catheter's down sides, there was a definite upside. I've had what I'd call a weak bladder for years. I wonder now if, or in what way, the cancer played into that. Was it cause or effect or simply coincidence? What ever the reason, I hadn't be able to sit through a movie in years. I was always the guy desperate for an isle seat, because I was going to have to take a break before it was over. I'd gotten very good at catching the lull just before the climax of a movie.

The same went for trips by car. I'd long since abandoned that male trait of not being the one to give in an ask to pull over. There were trees along Hwy 71 between Texarkana and Shreveport that sent me Christmas cards due to our intimacy. Now, suddenly, I found that with a bigger bag, I could go almost forever without the need of a bathroom break. I could take in a double feature or just blow a kiss to those familiar trees as I zoomed past. It was wonderful after so many years with my bladder calling the shots.

It got even better than just the endurance. The urine bag at my ankle was equipped with a valve and a drain hose. I didn't even have to find someplace private to offload. I could just step onto a storm drain or some other appropriate place, then bend down as though tying my shoe. I'd pull out the drain tube far enough to avoid splatter then open the valve. I could be in the middle of a parking lot or right along the sidewalk in front of a store. I didn't even have to step out of the car if I was on a trip. I'd just stick my leg out the door, deploy the tube, and open the valve. My super power was bionic urination.

I'm grateful for my new bladder. The upside of bionic urination didn't offset the downsides of the bags and tubes. But as wonderful as the new bladder is compared to the prospect of a life time with an ostomy bag, it is not my OEM (Original Equipment Manufacturer) bladder.

The original bladder was designed by the same guy who set the speed of light, and consisted of a ball of muscle surrounding a water tight sphere. My new bladder was made by some very smart and talented guys, but they were not omnipotent. They had to work with what they could find. They used a piece of my small intestine. Think sausage skin.

I learned an interesting thing about the small intestine. Interesting to me at least. It turns out that the small intestine is lined with a mucus membrane. It producers mucus. Your sinuses are also mucus membranes and produces similar, if not the same, mucus. So, my new bladder is full of boogers. Bladder boogers I call them. Urine soaked boogers that pass through my urethra when I urinate. I wonder how that will affect my next drug test.

As my new bladder was healing it was especially prolific in the production of mucus. There was also the occasional blood clot for the first week or so. Because the openings in the business end of the foley catheter is so small, it occasionally got clogged. I had to flush my healing bladder daily with sterile water. The hospital sent me home with a huge syringe and a bottle of the stuff.

I would attach the syringe to a port in the catheter and inject 55ccs of sterile water into my bladder. I could then use the syringe to suck it back out giving my new store bought bladder a good rinsing. I could see what had come back out of me through the clear syringe. It was disconcerting in those early days.

Now 55ccs is the same displacement of a small motor scooter engine. It didn't take long to run through the bottle of sterile water I'd brought home from the hospital. When I ran out of water, I hobbled out to the pharmacy to get some more. Imagine my surprise to learn that you need a prescription to get sterile water. I assumed that sterile water was just pure Dihydrogen Monoxide.

But parsing the words more carefully I realize that sterile mean lifeless, not pure. I wonder what is in "official" sterile water that makes it a controlled substance. Considering I was shooting 55ccs of it up into my body every day, I wanted to know. (*I have since learned that the prescription is to make sure that you get water sterile to medical standards, and so that you can claim it on your insurance.*)

— — —

The way I was wired up, or tubed up, when I left the hospital was that the ileal conduit was a shunt, catching the output of my kidneys. I can't get an image in my head of what it looked like inside of me. But in some way Dr. Henderson arranged it so that when the time came to remove them, all he had to do was snip a suture holding the tubes in place at the surface and pull them out.

A couple of days before my appointment for that procedure, I began to experience severe discomfort in my back. I first thought it was just muscle strain, but the discomfort graduated to outright pain over night. I called the clinic, and they moved my appointment up a day.

We already had plans for our other dear friends Bill and Denise Johnson to take me for this trip. Unfortunately moving it up a day meant Denise couldn't make it, so it was just me and Bill. Bill swung by, picked me up and we were on our way to Shreveport.

By now the discomfort had progressed through pain and had become outright agony. Bill is a pretty talkative fellow, but the gasping little breaths I was able to take only allowed answers of a syllable or two. He would later tell me that he was truly worried that I wouldn't make it to the clinic.

I don't remember much about that trip. Pain is all I recall. It was so intense that in the infrequent lulls, I'd fall almost instantly asleep until the next wave of pain hit. I eventually found my self sitting on an exam table while Dr. Henderson and another person looked me over. "The pain is your body telling you it's time to remove the shunts," Dr. Henderson explained.

He snipped the sutures and pulled the tubes out. That was a strange sensation. I could feel the tubes sliding through my body, almost as though a small mouse was running around inside of me. I had imagined the conduit running strait from my kidneys to the opening in my side, a distance of a few inches. The mouse was running a circle in my torso and the good doctor pulled a foot or more of tubing out of me. It must have been coiled inside of me.

The mouse running around inside of me was a strange sensation, but the biggest change was the instant cessation of the pain. It was like he flipped a switch and the pain was gone instantly. I was ecstatic. Bill was waiting for me in the lobby and couldn't believe the change that had come over me. I laughed and talked Bill's ears off on the way home. Bill says he's never seen such a change in a person in such a short time.

With the ostomy bag gone my convalesce speeded up. I don't recall the exact number of days that passed between the time the ileal conduit was removed, and I got rid of the catheter. Getting rid of the catheter wasn't easy as it had a nasty surprise waiting for us.

Sharon was with me on the day I was to have the catheter removed. The procedure is fairly straight forward. The bulb that holds the catheter in the bladder is filled with saline solution. It can be drained using a valve on the tubing still outside of my body. Once the fluid is released the bulb collapses and the catheter tube should pull right out.

Dr. Henderson drained the saline, then gave the tube a good yank. It just about lifted me off the table. It would not come out. It had surprised me so I had yelped pretty loud. The doctor seemed hesitant to go ahead a pull it out. I told him to ignore my vocalizations and just pull the damn thing out. He declined, explaining that he had already pulled as hard as he was comfortable pulling. "Any harder might do damage," he explained.

He wasn't sure why it wouldn't come out. One, hopefully remote, possibility was that a suture had gone through the tube while they were closing me up. The doctor didn't think that was the problem and it would turn out he was correct.

Our only real option at this point was to put me out and let the good doctor try to push a tool into my urethra between the catheter and my body to release what ever was stuck. He told me that if he couldn't free the tube that way, he might have to seek surgical remedy. That would be a major setback as I would then have to heal from having a very sensitive part of my body cut into. I wasn't crazy about the idea, but if that's what we had to do, then there there was nothing for it but to get it done.

Dr. Henderson was able to find an operating room at a different hospital downtown just three days later. In the mean time I went back home. Dr. Henderson told me that there was a small possibility that the tube might just fall out on its own and to let him know if that happened so that he could cancel the surgery. Three days later the darn thing was still stuck tight so Charles picked me up and we set off for Shreveport.

In the car, on the way over, I started to hurt. The pain increased until I was in agony by the time we got to the hospital. They checked me in and I once again found myself laying naked under a sheet surrounded by female nurses. That was the least of my worries by now because I was in so much pain, I would have welcomed the itch box at this point.

I was given a shot of something to relieve the pain. I don't remember exactly what it was. I don't think it was morphine, but it was powerful. It didn't help. I was eventually given at least one more injection, but I think maybe two.

I would later comment to Charles that the stuff had absolutely no effect on me. Charles laughed heartily and assured me that it had indeed had an effect. Apparently, between the waves of pain, I would go completely out. Then, when awake, what I remember as articulate descriptions of my discomfort were actually ramblings that might have well as been in a lost language.

They wheeled me into the operating room where Dr. Henderson was waiting. I think we again discussed the possibility of his having to surgically remove the tube. I was likely speaking in tongues so it's doubtful if we came to any useful decision.

I awakened, once again in the room I was in before the surgery. I looked at the attendant and asked her in an elegant and articulate manor about the surgery. She looked at me as though I was reciting the Jabberwocky by Lewis Carrol, then pushed my head down and told me to get some rest.

When I again came too, I felt quite awake — unlike the last time I came out of anesthesia. Dr. Henderson was there and I asked him if he was able to remove the catheter without surgery. He laughed and said that they never got me on the operating table. As they were maneuvering me to move me over, the catheter just fell out. It seems it had finally come loose. The pain I'd been experiencing was the end of the catheter scraping my urethra as it worked it's way out. If I'd just pulled it on out that morning, I might have avoided a lot more pain, the drugs, and a wasted trip to the OR. Looking back I'm certain I know what happened. Be warned, it's gross so skip the next three paragraphs if you're squeamish.

During the five weeks I had the catheter, it would allow leakage for a few days, then go dry for a few days. I can imagine the foley bulb nestling into the

the depression at the bottom of my new bladder where the sphincter is located, like a ping-pong ball in a funnel. Sometimes the seal would be tight, but other times it wasn't. Maybe the shape of the new bladder would change. For what ever reason, the bulb wouldn't seal completely allowing the contents of my bladder to seep out between the catheter tube and the wall of my urethra. The seepage consisted of urine of course, but also some of the mucus my new bladder produced.

For several days just before the first trip to remove the catheter, I had been dry. When the bulb again sealed, there were still globs of mucus trapped in my urethra, between the wall and the catheter. When they dried up, they glued the tube to my urethra. When Dr. Henderson collapsed the foley bulb, I began to seep again. The liquid eventually softened the dried mucus, freeing the catheter.

Dr. Henderson seemed somewhat skeptical of my hypothesis, but never offered another explication.

OK, it was a fight but the catheter was now gone and for the first time in more than five weeks, I didn't have any tubes sticking out of my body.

LIFE WITHOUT TUBES

The removal of the catheter brought its own challenges, namely incontinence. Severe incontinence. I'd been warned of this and had covered the passenger seat of the car with a trash bag. I laid a towel on top of that and topped the towel with a disposable bed pad. By the time we got home, the bed pad and towel were soaked, but the stack held long enough to keep the seat dry.

I was now in diapers. Yes, I know that the official name is "Adult Protective Undergarment." They were diapers. Big diaper, but still diapers. Having to wear diapers for a while wasn't even in the top twenty of ego adjusting experiences I'd had in the last five weeks, and I was in no mood to sugar coat the situation. For now, I was wearing diapers.

There were three possible outcomes. I might remain incontinent, I might eventually be unable to urinate on my own and require catheters, or I might regain complete bladder control. I had to strengthen the sphincter in my bladder. I began a series of exercises known as Kegel exercises. These are specifically designed to strengthen pelvic floor muscles and are used for several things including treating incontinence. It would be months before I would know how much control I'd eventually recover. So I'd be in diapers for at least a few months.

An adult in diapers is not the same as an infant in diapers. The adult bladder produces more liquid than any diaper can hope to contain. The purpose of these protective garments is to absorb leaks. In the first couple of weeks I wasn't leaking, I was pouring at a steady rate. I used paper towels as homemade sanitary napkins to argument the absorption capacity of the diapers. Even so, I had to change out about every two hours.

I carried a couple of small garbage bags with me, one filled with fresh paper towels and diapers, the other filled with diapers and paper towels that weren't fresh. Not fresh at all. You didn't want to be nearby when I opened it to deposit used material.

Just a few days later I was able to hold my bladder while sitting. Unfortunately, I would suffer a complete bladder dump as soon as I stood up. I found a jug with a lid that I could use to collect the contents of my bladder as I stood. This wasn't much of a problem at home. If I had guests, I'd just explain the problem and wait for them to leave the room before standing.

Just a week after losing the catheter, Dr. Henderson cleared me to return to work. I still had a couple of weeks of paid leave left, but decided that if I could function at work, I would go back and save the leave time in case I needed it later. This was only possible because I had my own office.

My office is in the pre-press production area, a relatively isolated part of the building. The people that work for me work evenings, so I had the place to myself for most of the day. I closed the blinds on the windows that look out onto the floor. I then closed my office door, though I didn't lock it. I made sure that everybody in the building was warned to not come into my office without knocking. I even put a sign on the door, warning that I would not be held responsible for any trauma resulting from an unannounced entry.

I should mention that the first chore facing me as I returned was awaiting me in my office. Approaching the door I noticed and xacto knife taped to the door just under a sign that read, "Welcome back. POP on in."

My employees had filled my office to a depth of about three feet with balloons. They were just higher than my desk. Our area is supplied with compressed air, so they didn't blow up all of those balloons by mouth. It took me an hour to pop enough to get to my desk. They saw how far I was from complete recovery and finished clearing them out for me overnight.

— — —

The surgery was in September of 2011. I kept getting better as time passed and January of 2012, I was very much recovered. I only needed dia .. uh adult protective undergarments at night. During the day I was back in regular clothing, though to this day I still use a homemade paper towel sanitary napkin.

It's easy to let something like this become an excuse for not doing anything, but I discovered that the more I pushed my self, the better I got. So, when our hot water heater finally gave up the ghost, I decided to replace it.

I was going to replace the rusted tank with a tankless water heater. The change in equipment meant significant plumbing as the wall mounted tankless unit would be in a slightly different position from the old tank.

I was able to get the unit I wanted locally. I actually went up in capacity because they had one in stock and I didn't have to pay shipping on it. Shipping would have made the smaller unit more expensive, so that was a no brainer. I brought it home and laid it down on a piece of cardboard, then drew out all of the connections and pipe I'd need. A quick trip to the hardware store and I was ready to go. I haven't sweated a lot of copper in my day so I was concerned about my plumbing, but my fears were unfounded.

One thing the instructions were adamant about was that the unit would require a minimum of a three-quarter inch gas line. Anything smaller, the paper work warned, and the unit would not even attempt to come on. It would simply warn that there was an insufficient gas supply. I checked and confirmed that the supply line to the old unit was three-quarter inch.

I did all of the pre-plumbing I could, then drained the old tank and pulled it out. I mounted the new unit to the wall and sweated the new copper over to the heater. Last of all I began to run the new gas line. Wow! It's amazing how similar a three-quarter inch fitting looks to a half-inch fitting.

Buy this time it was late and I couldn't even get to the store for material so I dragged that ragged old tank back into the house, set it in front of the new unit and used flex connections to run water to it from the new lines to get us through the night.

I climbed under the house and found where the half-inch black pipe tied into the one-inch main line. I bought the material I needed the next morning and ran a new one-inch line all the way back to the new unit. A few hours later I took a long soak with an endless supply of hot water.

It wasn't just that I now had the best water heater I'd ever owned, but I'd done it myself, much as I would have before the surgery. The job had required a lot of straining and effort. In addition to plumbing the water lines, I'd climbed under the house to replace black pipe gas lines. I felt as though I was well on the way back to my old self.

By the summer of 2012, I was almost back to my old self. I don't think I ever completely recovered, never quite reached a hundred percent. But I got close, at least ninety percent. We were riding motorcycles with our friends again. The only concession was that I continued to sleep in protective garments and kept a bed pad on the bed at night. I was again tackling jobs by myself that had my kids concerned. Truly, a sign of progress.

Our house was built in 1898. It's a large two story with a full attic. It also has a balcony over the front porch that is a more recent addition. The front is an unsupported span of about twenty-four feet. This makes for a great front porch with an open view. We love the balcony and eat out there when the weather is good. Unfortunately, the flat floor of the balcony had developed leaks and over the years, water damaged the stringer supporting front edge of the balcony.

The original stringer was three two-by-sixes scabbed together. The rest of the house is cedar, but this newer addition was white pine and quite susceptible to water damage. By October of 2014, the front edge of the balcony was sagging noticeably and the floor felt springy as you walked on the balcony. It was time to do something.

I checked several salvage places and found a large industrial I-beam that was twenty-three feet long, six inches wide and six-teen inches tall. I paid scrap metal price of forty-four cents per pound for it and a couple of eight foot long four by four steel posts.

The first challenge was getting the twenty-three foot long, four hundred pound I-beam home. I've got a six-teen foot trailer with a tall tail gate. I had the guys at the salvage yard use their forklift to put it on the trailer. I tied the tail gate to the beam to keep it from dragging then headed out. I had to assure the guys at the salvage yard I wouldn't hold them responsible if the beam damaged my trailer. I could see them shaking their heads as I pulled out of the yard.

I got the thing home and managed to get it unloaded from the trailer. It stretched from the gate to the steps to the porch. That was the easy part part. Now I was going to have to remove the old stringer, build a temporary support for the balcony, then lift the new one almost fifteen feet from the ground into place.

To put it simply, none of my friends or coworkers believed that I could do it by myself. People kept asking me who I was going to get to do it for me, then meet me with skepticism when I explained that I would do it myself. A few would ask if I were going to rent a crane or lift. I would have, but there were several permanent fixtures in the front yard that would have to have come out. I decided it was just easier to do it by hand. This was universally met with complete disbelief. The only exceptions were Sharon and the kids. They would just shrug their shoulders and say, "If he said he'll do it himself, he'll do it himself."

I used pipes to roll the thing as close as I could to the porch. Obviously I didn't bench press the thing into place, it weighed four-hundred pounds. I could lift one end a couple of inches and Mrs. Sharon would stuff cribbing under that end. We'd go to the the other end, I'd lift it and she would stuff cribbing under it. Go back and repeat. After a little more than an hour, it was high enough to set on the platforms at the side of the front steps.

My incontinence was greatly improved, but the strain of lifting that beam was testing my control. If my bladder wasn't almost completely empty, the strain would cause a leak. I had to run the the bathroom at least once every hour to keep things manageable.

Once the beam was on the platforms I could restart the stack of cribbing, reducing it's hight and making it less precarious. The second lift, from the platforms to the top of the pedestals on which the support columns would sit was about five feet. I was still making each lift by hand with Mrs. Sharon adding the cribbing.

The lifts from the ground to the platforms and from the platforms to the top of the pedestals required me to steady the beam by hand. The sixteen inch tall, six inch wide piece of metal was top heavy and the cribbing wasn't steady. I also had to move the beam sideways into position on the last move of each lift. That required moving the beam by hand.

Once the beam was on the pedestal, it was directly beneath its final position and the last lift of six feet was was straight up. I was able to replace the muscles and profanity method of lifting with one that used hydraulic bottle jacks. I built runners running on both side of the beam up to the deck. It was now caught between two-by-fours and guided into place. I used a bottle jack to raise each end a few inches then nail a brace in place.

The security camera at the front door captured

the final rise and I was able to make a stop motion video of that last lift. It condenses the final six hour lift to about thirty-seconds The video is still available on line.

http://www.guywheatley.com/gifs/BeamLift.gif.

Fixing the balcony not only improved the house, it signified my recovery. That project made me feel that I was finally back close to the man I was before the cancer.

LIFE AFTER CANCER

Six years after having my bladder replaced I'm grateful for every second. I remember that horrible Friday afternoon on the mezzanine at work, trying to come to grips with the idea that I might not have much longer.

I think I would have come to grips with however much time I had left. Fortunately, I didn't have to find out. I've had six birthday's since then, six Christmases and six Thanksgivings. I've had countless hugs and kisses from my wife and children. We bought a convertible and I gave the Valkyrie to Brandon. It looks so much better at his house than smashed at the bottom of a ravine. The six years I've been given are a gift of immeasurable treasure.

I have a hard time thinking of myself as a cancer survivor. I never suffered the ravages of chemotherapy or radiation. I never lost my hair or spent hours suffering the bone deep pain of drugs to increase white blood cell count. I didn't spend hours hugging the toilet and lose weight because I couldn't eat or keep food down. I had it pretty easy. I had an operation that kept me in the hospital for about seven days, then spent a few months recovering. Hardly the ordeal a diagnosis of cancer normally heralds.

Five years later, my daughter would not be so fortunate. Her fight with cancer would last a year and she would suffer the pain and indignities that I escaped. Praise God that as of this writing, she has completed her treatment and is cancer free. But watching her fight made me realize how fortunate I really was. The courage and grace with which she faced her ordeal make me proud, and I wonder how close I would have come to her courage.

Cancer changes so many things with its appearance. You will never think of your body the same way again. Certainly in my case, a complacency was gone. I know there are things in the world that will try to kill me, accidents, viruses, dangerous animals. But this was different. This was from within my own body. A killer that was not merely inside of me, but actually a part of me. This wasn't me and my body fighting the world, this was part of my body threatening my life.

My survival is due to the determination and brilliance of the medical community in fighting this disease. Dr. Henderson questioned me, trying to find something that might have triggered my cancer. I would occasionally smoke a few cigarillos on weekend rides. Four of five times a year I'd get a box of six. There is no way to know for sure, but I doubt my tobacco use was a factor. Even so, I haven't smoked one since.

I was lucky in so many ways, not the least was the medical community with whom I went through this ordeal. Dr. Henderson was wonderful, inspiring confidence, supporting, and patient. He told me that both Sharon and I were approaching this with good attitudes. He encouraged and help me with my attitude with humor and warmth. He gave me many words of wisdom and good advice, but one thing he repeated several times will stick with me the rest of my life, "Listen to your body. It will tell you what it needs and when it's having a problem." He always patiently listened to me, taking in my observations as he diagnosed my progress.

Another fortunate placement was being at Christus Schumpert Highland. I've been a patient in a couple of other hospitals and have visited friends and relatives in the hospital many times. I've never felt as cared for as I did during this stay. I don't recall having to wait more than a couple of minutes the few times I pressed the call button. I could count on somebody checking on me almost every hour even though I hadn't called anybody. From bringing us ice to providing a bed for Sharon, they made my stay better in a thousand little ways. They acted as much like concerned friends as medical professionals.

Let me end this with advice for anybody facing this disease and their family. Attitude is crucial. I believe a good attitude will increase you odds by encouraging your body to fight. At the very least, it helps to not be depressed.

Wave goodby to your former concept of dignity. You do things and have things done to you that are decidedly undignified by most peoples understanding. I came to understand that real dignity isn't defined by what happens to you, but how you respond to those things.

Keep your chin up, keep a good attitude, and don't lose your since of humor. Laugh at the funny things, no matter how undignified they are. Laugh every chance you get.

I was lucky and I get to look back on this from six-years later, but I was cognizant that those might have been my last weeks with my loved ones. I wanted to leave them with as many good memories as I could. I didn't want their last memories of me to be of somebody depressed and in pain.

My biggest regret of the time was that I was leaving Sharon with less than stellar financial prospects. I didn't have a lot of insurance and we'd borrowed against that. Our meager savings quickly evaporated in the face of our combined medical expenses. I'm still trying to fix that. I hope that my writing will provide at least some additional income.

My last piece of advice is for the family. Even though your loved one is facing a personal challenge, their love for you hasn't died. They will try to protect you by putting on a brave face. Don't challenge their effort. It's the last thing they can do for you and it comes from a place of love.

ABOUT THE AUTHOR

Guy Wheatley grew up as a military dependent living on or near military bases until age thirteen. He started junior high school in his family hometown of Gillett Arkansas where his father taught him to hunt and fish. He played football in high school and held farm related jobs during the summers throughout high school and college. He also spent one summer as deck crew on a Mississippi River tow boat.

Leaving college before graduating, he took a job running an insurance agency for Planters and Merchants Bank in Gillett. Two years later he took up the same position for Merchants and Planters Bank in Hughes, Arkansas, just about 45 minutes east of Memphis Tennessee.

He had been doing freelance editorial cartoons for several years and eventually took a job with the Texarkana Gazette as an editorial artist. His interest in technology led him to be an early adopter of computers in the newsroom where he became "The computer guy."

Eventually he moved from graphics to technology and is currently the Technical Services Administrator at the Texarkana Gazette. During this time he went back to school and received his BAAS degree with a concentration in English at Texas A&M – Texarkana.

He is an avid reader but has also contributed several articles and columns to the Gazette throughout his career. He also wrote the "Texarkana Bikers Blog," a motorcycle blog, for the paper.

Other Books by Guy B Wheatley

The Time I'm Given:
The first book in this series where we meet Zee and Zack for the first time as they struggle to secure Zee's humanity.
The Time I'm Given — Available on Amazon

The Name I'm Given:
The sequel to *The Time I'm Given*.
Available on Amazon in paper back and for Kindle and other e-readers.
The Name I'm Given — Available on Amazon

Doubt:
A short story, available at no charge as PDF
Doubt — A short story

The Life I'm Given:
Emily takes up the narrative in the third offering from this world. She returns to her home town and has her daughter buried close to her parents. While on this voyage of self discovery, she takes on the task of saving a local girl and winds up in the city of Hot Springs. The fight takes place in the secret tunnels under the down town area, a hold out from the Hot Springs gangster era.
The Life I'm Given — Available on Amazon